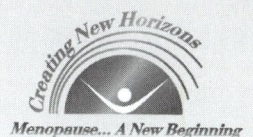

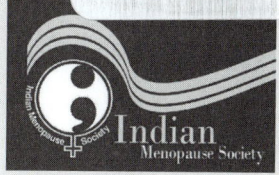

1000 Multiple Choice Questions on

Menopause

1000 Multiple Choice Questions on

Menopause

Editor

Suvarna Khadilkar MD, DGO, FICOG, CIMP,
PG Diploma in Endocrinology (South Wales UK)
President IMS 2017–18
Consultant Gynecologist and Endocrinologist
Bombay Hospital and Medical Research Center, Mumbai
Professor and Head
Department of Obstetrics and Gynecology
Government Medical College, Kolhapur, Maharashtra, India, Till April (2013)
Chairperson
Endocrinology Committee FOGSI 2011–13
Editor-In-Chief
Journal of Obstetrics and Gynecology of India
Treasurer
Federation of Obstetrics and Gynecology of India

Co-editors

Seema Sharma MS, FICMCH, MICOG, FMAS
Professor and Unit Head
Obstetrics and Gynaecology MGMCH, Jaipur
Secretary General Elect IMS
Vice President, Elect JOGS, NARCHI, Rajasthan
Ex-Chairperson, Exam Committee IMS

Punit Bhojani MS, DNB, FCPS, DGO, DFP
Consultant Obstetrician and Gynecologist,
Mumbai
attached to Surya,
Kohinoor and Global Hospitals
Member of Managing Council of MOGS

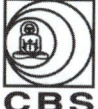

CBS

CBS Publishers and Distributors Pvt Ltd

New Delhi • Bengaluru • Chennai • Kochi • Kolkata • Mumbai
Bhopal • Bhubaneswar • Hyderabad • Jharkhand • Nagpur • Patna • Pune • Uttarakhand • Dhaka (Bangladesh)

1000 Multiple Choice Questions on

Menopause

ISBN: 978-93-88178-83-9

Scientific content, art work and publishing
Copyright © Indian Menopause Society, Editor, and Publisher

First Edition: 2019

Published by Satish Kumar Jain and produced by Varun Jain for

CBS Publishers and Distributors Pvt Ltd

4819/XI Prahlad Street, 24 Ansari Road, Daryaganj, New Delhi 110 002, India.
Ph: 23289259, 23266861, 23266867   Fax: 011-23243014
Website: www.cbspd.com   e-mail: delhi@cbspd.com; cbspubs@airtelmail.in.

Corporate Office: 204 FIE, Industrial Area, Patparganj, Delhi 110 092, India
Ph: 4934 4934   Fax: 4934 4935   e-mail: publishing@cbspd.com; publicity@cbspd.com

Branches

- **Bengaluru:** Seema House 2975, 17th Cross, K.R. Road, Banasankari 2nd Stage, Bengaluru 560 070, Karnataka, India
  Ph: +91-80-26771678/79   Fax: +91-80-26771680   e-mail: bangalore@cbspd.com
- **Chennai:** 7, Subbaraya Street, Shenoy Nagar, Chennai 600 030, Tamil Nadu, India.
  Ph: +91-44-26680620, 26681266   Fax: +91-44-42032115   e-mail: chennai@cbspd.com
- **Kochi:** 42/1325, 1326, Power House Road, Opposite KSEB Power House, Ernakulam 682 016, Kochi, Kerala, India.
  Ph: +91-484-4059061-65   Fax: +91-484-4059065   e-mail: kochi@cbspd.com
- **Kolkata:** 6/B, Ground Floor, Rameswar Shaw Road, Kolkata-700 014 (West Bengal), India.
  Ph: +91-33-2289-1126, 2289-1127, 2289-1128   e-mail: kolkata@cbspd.com
- **Mumbai:** 83-C, Dr E Moses Road, Worli, Mumbai-400018, Maharashtra, India.
  Ph: +91-22-24902340/41   Fax: +91-22-24902342   e-mail: mumbai@cbspd.com

Representatives

Bhopal	0-8319310552	**Bhubaneswar**	0-9911037372	**Hyderabad**	0-9885175004
Jharkhand	0-9811541605	**Nagpur**	0-9421945513	**Patna**	0-9334159340
Pune	0-9623451994	**Uttarakhand**	0-9716462459	**Dhaka (Bangladesh)**	01912-003485

Printed at: JS Offset, Patparganj Industiral Area, Delhi-110092

Foreword

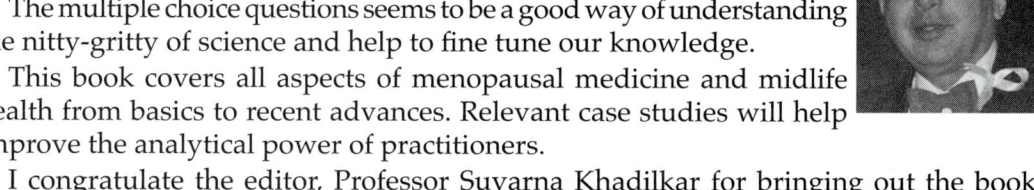

*Me*nopause and midlife health are surrounded by controversies and new concepts and protocols have been reported in recent literature.

The multiple choice questions seems to be a good way of understanding the nitty-gritty of science and help to fine tune our knowledge.

This book covers all aspects of menopausal medicine and midlife health from basics to recent advances. Relevant case studies will help improve the analytical power of practitioners.

I congratulate the editor, Professor Suvarna Khadilkar for bringing out the book which fulfils a long-standing demand. I appreciate the hard work put in by the editor and compliment her. I am sure that this book will be a good reference book and will be of great help to postgraduates students appearing for various diploma and degree courses, such as MRCPI, MRCOG, FRCOG, common entrance exams. This book will also be useful for medical teachers and doctors who are focusing on menopausal medicine in their day-to-day practice.

CN Purandare

MD, MA Obst. (IRL), DGO, DFP
DOBST RCPI (Dublin), FRCOG (UK), FRCPI (Ireland)
FACOG (USA), FAMS, FICOG, FICMCH, PGD MLS (Law)
Consultant Obstetrician and Gynecologist

President FIGO
Dean, Indian College of Obstetricians and Gynaecologists
President, FOGSI (2009)
President, Indian College of OBGYN (2009)
Editor Emeritus Journal-FOGSI
Ex Hon Professor OBGYN, Grant Medical College and
JJ Hospital, Mumbai
Hon Consultant, Mumbai Police
Hon Consultant, Saifee Hospital and BSES Hospital, Mumbai
Visiting Consultant, St Elizabeth Hospital Mumbai

Preface

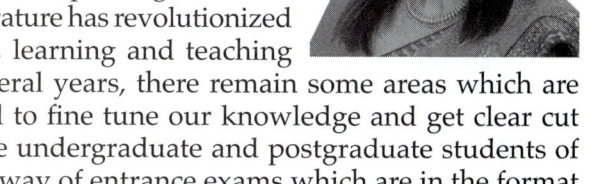

*I*t gives me great pleasure to present to you this unique book *1000 Multiple Choice Questions on Menopause*. Indian menopause society is a large organization of over 3000 members, 43 societies across the length and breadth of India, achieving new heights every year. Our society is dedicated to improving health of menopausal women.

Practising menopausal medicine needs updating of knowledge from time to time as the recent literature has revolutionized many concepts. In spite of practising, learning and teaching various aspects of menopause for several years, there remain some areas which are not very well understood. So we need to fine tune our knowledge and get clear cut answers to unanswered questions. The undergraduate and postgraduate students of today have several hurdles to clear by way of entrance exams which are in the format of MCQs, enabling objective assessment.

So we at IMS undertook this project of 1000 MCQs which will cover and touch upon all aspects of menopausal medicine and also midlife health. Many of the IMS members have contributed to this book with a great enthusiasm. I appreciate efforts of each one of them. The correct answers given in the book may not necessarily be the ideal answers, but are the most appropriate choices from the given options. These simulate some practice situations where the most ideal treatment may not be available and then you need to choose from the available options. I sincerely hope that this book helps all those who have passion to improvise the knowledge to perfection from examination as well as the practice point of view!

I thank all the contributors for providing the chapters without any disclosure to make. My co-editors Seema Sharma and Punit Bhojani have worked very hard to make this endeavour possible. I sincerely thank reviewers specially Meeta, Jyothi, Ranu and Ambuja for sparing their valuable time.

I will put on record my sincere appreciation of Mr Ramesh Krishnamachari of CBS Publishers and Distributors (P) Ltd. for assisting in the editorial process efficiently and promptly.

The tremendous amount of love, support and appreciation I received from the entire IMS family has been the continuous source of inspiration for me to do more and more quality work. I thank IMS family for being there.

Long Live IMS

Suvarna Khadilkar

Suvarna Khadilkar

Contributors

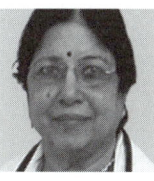

Ambuja Choranur
MD, DGO
Former Professor and Head
Department of
Obstetrics & Gynecology
Osmania Medical College
Hyderabad, Telangana
Visiting Professor
Saveetha University Chennai
Faculty for National Board of Examinations
New Delhi

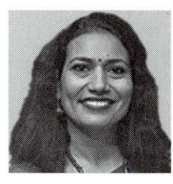

Jyoti Jaiswal
MBBS, MD (Obs & Gyne), FMAS, CIMP
Professor and Unit Head
Department of Obstetrics &
Gynecology
Pt. JNM Medical College
Raipur (CG)
Chairperson, Medical Education Committee
IMS, India
Chapter Secretary IMS, Raipur, (2014-2017)

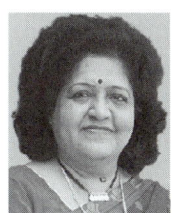

Ashwini Bhalerao-Gandhi
MD, DGO, DFP, FCPS, DNB, FICOG
Consultant Gynecologist
PD Hinduja Hospital, Mumbai

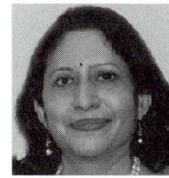

Kanchan Sortey
MD, FICMCH
Consultant Gynecologist
Infertologist, Endoscopic Surgeon
Director
Sortey Hospital and
Research Centre

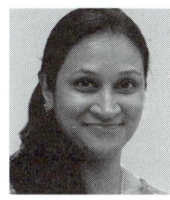

Bhumika
MBBS, DGO, DNB (Obs & Gyne),
MNAMS
Consultant, Saifee Hospital
Masina Hospital
St Elizabeth Hospital
Apollo Spectra Hospital
Mumbai

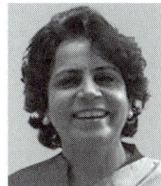

Kawita Bapat   MS, FICOG
Director
One Centre for
Gynecological Excellence
Senior Practicing
(Obstetrics and gynecology)
Bapat Hospital, Indore

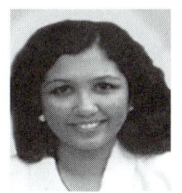

Deepali Prakash Kale
MBBS, DGO (MUHS), DGO (CPS),
FCPS, DNBE, FMAS (WALS)
Assistant Professor
Department of
Obstetrics & Gynecology
Nowrosjee Wadia Maternity
Hospital & Seth G.S. Medical College, Mumbai

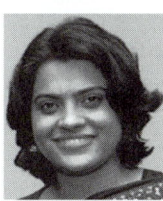

Madhuri Mehendale
MBBS, DGO, FCPS, DNB
Assistant Professor
Department of
Obstetrics & Gynecology
Lokmanya Tilak Municipal
Medical College Mumbai

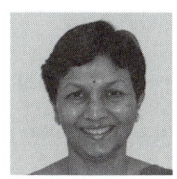

Jyothi Unni
FRCOG (UK)
Head
Department of Obstetrics &
Gynecology
Jehangir Hospital, Pune

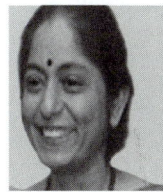

Meeta
MBBS, MD (Obs & Gyne)
Co-director, Consultant
Obstetrics & Gynecology
Tanvir Hospital, Hyderabad
President 2012
Indian Menopause Society

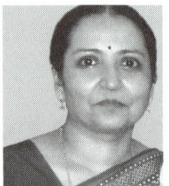

Navneet Takkar
Associate Professor
Department of
Obstetrics & Gynecology
Government Medical College
& Hospital
Chandigarh

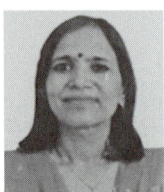

Neelam Aggarwal
Additional Professor
Department of
Obstetrics & Gynecology
PGIMER, Chandigarh

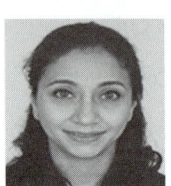

Preeti Deshpande
MS (Obs & Gyne)
Consultant Obstetrician and
Gynecologist
Guru Nanak Hospital, Bandra
Raheja-Fortis Hospital, Mahim
Mata Lachmi Hospital, Sion
Sambhav—Dr Preeti Deshpande's Clinic Wadala
Honorary Consultant
Sion Ayurvedic Hospital and College, Sion

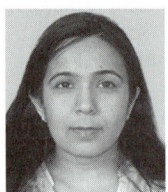

Priya Vora/Thakur
DNBE, DGO, FCPS, DFP, MBBS
Consultant
Dr. Vora's Gynecology
and Maternity Hospital
Bhatia Hospital,
Saint Elizabeth,
Ruxmani Lying–In Hospital
Mumbai

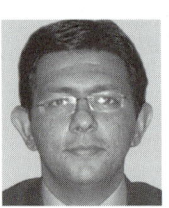

Punit Bhojani
MS, DNB, FCPS, DGO, DFP
Consultant
Obstetrician and Gynecologist
at Surya, Kohinoor & Global
Hospitals, Mumbai
Member, Managing
Council of MOGS

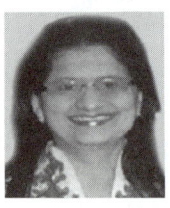

Rashmi Shah
Consultant Gynecologist
SRL Diagnostics
Jankharia Imaging Centre
Mumbai
IMS Patron
Mumbai Chapter
Treasurer & Joint Secretary
IMS India
Founder Editor
Journal of Midlife Health

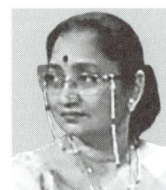

Seema Sharma
MS, FICMCH, MICOG, FMAS
Professor
Department of Obstetrics and
Gynecology
Mahatma Gandhi University of
Medical Sciences & Technology
Jaipur, Rajasthan

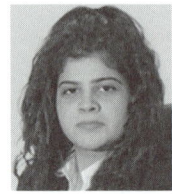

Shefali Kamal Kumar
Registered Dietitian and
Clinical Psychologist
Shefali Kumar's Health Mantr
Magnum Life Sciences Pvt Ltd

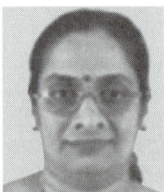

Shobana Mohan Das
Consultant Gynecologist and
Laparoscopic Surgeon
Sun Medical Centre
Thrissur, Kerala

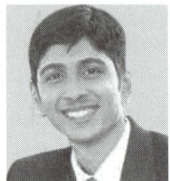

Siddesh Iyer
MBBS, DGO, DNB (Obs
& Gyne), MRCOG
Assistant Professor
Department of
Obstetrics and Gynecology
HBT Medical College and
Dr RN Cooper Municipal General Hospital
Mumbai

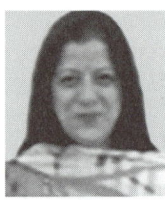

Sudha Sharma
Professor
Department of Obstetrics and
Gynecology
Government Medical
College, Jammu

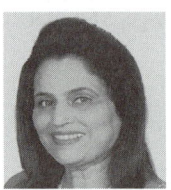

Suvarna Khadilkar
MD DGO FICOG, CIMP PG
Diploma in Endocrinology
(South Wales UK)
Consultant Endocrinologist and
Gynecologist
Bombay Hospital and Medical
Research Centre, Mumbai
President, IMS 2017

Contents

Abbreviations

ACOG:	American College of Obstetricians and Gynaecologists	MDPA:	Medroxy progesterone
AMH:	Anti-müllerian hormone	MHPG:	3 Methoxy–4 hydroxyphenylglycol
BMD:	Bone mineral density	MHT:	Menopausal hormone therapy
BRCA:	Breast cancer antigen	MHT:	Menopause hormone therapy
CABG:	Coronary artery bypass grafting	NAMS:	North American Menopause Society
CEE:	Conjugated equine estrogen	NSAIDs:	Non-steroidal anti-inflammatory drugs
CIN:	Cervical intraepithelial lesions		
COC:	Combined oral contraceptive	PEARL:	PGL4001 (ulipristal acetate) efficacy assessment in reduction of symptoms due to uterine leiomyomata
CSF:	Cerebrospinal fluid		
CVD:	Cardiovascular disease		
DEXA:	Dual energy X-ray absorptiometry		
DHEA:	Dehydroepiandrosterone	PEPI:	Postmenopausal estrogen progestin interventions
DMPA:	Depot medroxy progesterone acetate		
		POMC:	Pro-opiomelanocortin
ELITE:	Early versus late intervention trial with estradiol	POP:	Pelvic organ prolapse
		PRT:	Progressive resistance training
ELITT:	Endometrial laser intrauterine thermal therapy	SERM:	Selective estrogen receptor modulator
EPT:	Estrogen-progestin therapy	SHBG:	Sex hormone binding globulin
ESHRE:	European Society of Human Reproduction and Embryology	SPRM:	Selective progesterone receptor modulator.
FMD:	Flow–mediated dilation	STEAR:	Selective tissue estrogenic activity regulator
FNA:	Fine needle aspiration		
FPG:	Fasting plasma glucose	STRAW:	Stages of reproductive aging workshop
FSH:	Follicle stimulating hormone		
HDL:	High density lipoprotein	SUI:	Stress urinary incontinence
HERS:	Heart and estrogen/ progestin replacement study	SWAN:	Study of women health across the nation
HMB:	Heavy menstrual bleeding	TBEA:	Thermal balloon endometrial ablation
HNPCC:	Hereditary non-polyposis colonic cancer		
		TOT:	Transobturator tape
HSIL:	High grade squamous intraepithelial lesions	TSH:	Thyroid stimulating hormone
		TVT:	Tension free vaginal tape
ISD:	Intrinsic sphincter deficiency	WDHA	
IUCD:	Intrauterine contraceptive device	SYNDROME:	Watery diarrhea, hypokalemia, and achlorhydria syndrome
KEEPS:	Kronos early estrogen prevention study		
LDL:	Low density lipoproteins	WISE:	Women's ischemia syndrome evaluation
LSIL:	Low grade squamous intraepithelial lesions		

Editors thank FOGSI and editor for permitting us to reproduce some of the MCQs from the book "*Menopause, Current Concepts, 2004*", Editor CN Purandare/Associate editor SS Khadilkar. —A FOGSI Publication.

Chapter

1

Physiology of Menopause

◼ *Seema Sharma*

1. The rate of decline of hormones during menopause is:
   A. Variable
   B. Logarithmic
   C. Constant
   D. Biphasic

2. First pass metabolism of oral estrogen is associated with all of the following except:
   A. Increased synthesis of tri-glycerides
   B. Decreased synthesis of transcortin (costisole binding protein)
   C. Increased synthesis of sex hormone binding globulin
   D. Increased synthesis of angiotensinogen

3. Omics technologies have provided evidence that estrogen and intestinal microbiology can collectively influence all in postmenopausal women except:
   A. Obesity
   B. Diabetes
   C. Cancers
   D. Fall in vision

4. Postmenopausal women are more susceptible to all except:
   A. Fat redistribution
   B. Dyslipidemia
   C. Weight loss
   D. Osteopenia

5. Following the arrest of estradiol secretion by ovaries at menopause, all estrogens in postmenopausal women are made locally in peripheral target tissue according to physiological mechanisms of intracrinology.
   A. True
   B. False

6. STRAW staging of reproductive aging is based on which reference point:
   A. Appearance of symptoms of menopausal transition
   B. Menstrual irregularity
   C. Serum levels of estrogen, FSH and progesterone
   D. Date of final menstrual period

7. The highest incidence of an ovulatory cycles is the age of:
   A. 20–30 years
   B. 30–40 years
   C. 40 years and above
   D. None of the above

8. Phytoestrogens aglycons have higher affinity for following estrogen receptors:
   A. α
   B. β
   C. Both A and B
   D. None of the above

9. ER-α receptors are present in abundance in:
   A. Uterus
   B. Breast
   C. Vagina
   D. All of the above

10. Which of the following have only ER-α present?
    A. Liver
    B. Lungs
    C. Bones
    D. Uterus

11. ER-α receptors are present in abundance in:
    A. Liver-hepatocytes
    B. Adreneal–Zona glomerulosa
    C. Adrenal–Zona reticularis
    D. Lungs

12. ER-β receptors are present Predominantly in all except:
    A. Neurons
    B. Thyroid glands
    C. Medulla oblongata
    D. Liver

13. ER-β receptors are expressed in all expect:
    A. Heart
    B. Lungs
    C. Pons
    D. Hippocampus

14. Both ER-α and ER-β receptors are present in abundance in all except:
    A. Thyroid glands
    B. Pituitary gland
    C. Urinary bladder
    D. Breast
    E. Adrenal Zona Fasiculata

15. Ovarian tissue contents:
    A. Predominantly ER α receptors
    B. Predominantly ER β receptors
    C. Both A and B
    D. None of above

16. Vaginal cytological examination of postmenopausal women commonly exhibits:
    A. Majority of superficial cells
    B. Majority of intermediate cells
    C. Tadpole like cells
    D. Mainly basal and parabasal cells

17. JF Friess compression of morbidity concepts indicates:
    A. Postponing the illness to a short period of time just before death
    B. Preponing the illness during childhood
    C. Compressing morbidity during reproductive years
    D. None of the above

18. The years prior to menopause that encompass the change from normal ovulatory cycles to cassation of menses are known as:
    A. Climacteric
    B. Perimenopausal transition
    C. Premature menopause
    D. Menopause

19. Menopause occurs when the number of remaining follicles falls below a critical threshold regardless of age that number is:
    A. 40
    B. 5000
    C. 1000
    D. 4000

20. The average age of menopause (in India) according to Indian epidemiological studies is:
    A. 40 years
    B. 55.1 years
    C. 51.2 years
    D. 46 years

21. The affinity of estriol for estrogen receptors as compared to estradiol is:
    A. 5–10%
    B. 20–30%
    C. 45–55%
    D. 65–75%

22. An average woman may experience about _____ ovulatory events during her reproductive lifetime:
    A. 50
    B. 400
    C. 1000
    D. 4000

23. According to SWAN (Study of Women Health Across the Nation) study an earlier age of menopause is associated with all of the following except:
    A. Current smoking
    B. Lower education
    C. Lower socioeconomic status
    D. Prior use of oral contraceptives

24. 1–3 years after menopause serum FSH levels:
    A. Rise by 10–20 fold
    B. Rise 3 fold
    C. Decreases to minimum
    D. Reduces to half

25. 1–3 years after menopause serum LH levels:
    A. Rise by 10–20 fold
    B. Rise 3 fold
    C. Decreases to minimum
    D. Reduces to half

26. Rise in SLH levels posmenopausally is less pronounced than the FSH because:
    A. LH has a short half-life
    B. FSH has a specific negative feedback peptide like inhibin
    C. Both A and B are true
    D. None of the above

27. Postmenopausal ovary secretes:
    A. Androstenedione and estrogen
    B. Androstenedion and testosterone
    C. Estrogen and testosterone
    D. None of the above

28. Androstenedione circulating in blood of postmenopausal women:
    A. Is half that seen in premenopausal women
    B. Is derived mainly from adrenal gland
    C. Is only partly from ovary
    D. All of the above are correct

29. After menopause testosterone production decreases by approximately:
    A. 25%
    B. 10%
    C. 75%
    D. No change at all

30. A decade after menopause circulating levels of DHEA are:
    A. 70% less than in young adult life
    B. Same as in immediate postmenopausal phase
    C. Doubled than levels in young women
    D. None of the above

31. The circulating estradiol levels in postmenopausal women are:
    A. 100–200 pg/ml
    B. 10–20 pg/ml
    C. Nil
    D. 50 pg/ml

32. Postmenopausal production of estrogen is 45 mg/24 hours which is derived from:
    A. Secretion from ovaries
    B. Peripheral conversion of androstenedione
    C. Both A and B
    D. None of the above

33. Aromatization of androgens to estrogen:
    A. Is limited to adipose tissue only
    B. Is only documented in bone breast
    C. Is documented in almost every tissue
    D. All of the above

34. Mild hirsutism seen at perimeno-pausal age is due to:
    A. Genetic influence
    B. Increased androgen: estrogen ratio
    C. None of the above
    D. Both A and B

35. Neuroendocrine changes in meno-pausal age group are implicated for:
    A. Hot flushes and night sweats
    B. Sleep disturbances
    C. Mood disturbances
    D. Memory and cognition
    E. All of the above

36. Estrogen leads to following effect on levels of high density lipoprotein (HDL):
    A. Decrease
    B. Increase
    C. Remain the same
    D. Effect is variable

37. Premenopausal age group of women have:
    A. Lower LDL cholesterol
    B. Higher LDL cholesterol
    C. Lower HDL cholesterol
    D. None of the above

38. Postmenopausal age group of women have:
    A. Lower LDL cholesterol
    B. Higher HDL cholesterol
    C. Increased LDL cholesterol
    D. No changes in lipid profile

39. Every year spongy bone is remodeled by:
    A. 10%
    B. 25%
    C. 35%
    D. 40%

40. According to the recent data. Which is the main hormonal event that charac-terises early menopausal transition?
    A. Low oestrogen and high proges-terone level
    B. High FSH concentration and   bw AMH

C. FSH constantly > 25 IU/L
    D. AMH, inhibin B begin to decrease, estrogen level is still be normal, with erratic level of FSH and progesterone

41. These are causes of delayed meno-pause except:
    A. Multi parity
    B. Prior use of contraceptives
    C. Japanese race/ethnicity
    D. Decreased BMI

42. The symptoms related to decreasing follicular competence and then estrogen loss are:
    A. Cessation of normal menstruation or infrequent menses
    B. Vasomotor instability
    C. Urogenital atrophy
    D. Health problems secondary to long-term estrogen deprivation such as osteoporosis and cardio-vascular disease
    E. All of the above

43. All of the following affect age at meno-pause:
    A. Smoking
    B. Genetic menopause
    C. Surgery on ovaries
    D. Socioeconomic status
    E. All of the above.

44. In a 60 kg healthy postmenopausal woman the percentage of body water remains:
    A. 20–30%
    B. 45%
    C. 55%
    D. 75%

45. Amount of water that is used by body's fluid regulatory and cardio-vascular system to control fluid intake and output, thirst blood pressure is:
    A. 3–4 lit
    B. 10–12 lit
    C. 15–16 lit
    D. 20–25 lit

46. Resistance training has been found associated all with except:
  A. Increased muscle mass
  B. Improved insulin sensitivity
  C. Increased BMI
  D. Increased glucose transport

47. Addition of progesterone to estrogen replacement benefits
  A. Endometrium
  B. Breast
  C. Heart
  D. All of the above

Answer Key

1. A	10. A	19. C	28. D	37. A	46. C
2. B	11. A	20. D	29. A	38. C	47. A
3. D	12. D	21. B	30. A	39. C	
4. C	13. D	22. B	31. B	40. D	
5. A	14. A	23. D	32. B	41. D	
6. D	15. C	24. A	33. C	42. E	
7. C	16. D	25. B	34. B	43. E	
8. B	17. A	26. C	35. E	44. C	
9. D	18. B	27. B	36. B	45. A	

References

1. **A** Barbo DM. The Physiology of the menopause. *Med. Clin North Am.* 1987.
4. **C** Chen KL, et al. Estrogens and female liver health. Steroids, 2018 May; 33:38–43.
5. **A** Labrie F, et al. Science of intracrinology in postmenopausal women. menopause 2017, June; 24(6):702–12.
6. **B** Sióbán D Harlow, et al. Executive summary of Straw+10: Addressing the Unfinished Agenda of Staging Reproductive Aging Climacteric. 2012 Apr; 15(2): 105–14.
8-15. Morito K, et al. Interaction of phytoestrogens with estrogen receptor X and B. *Biol Pharm bull.* 2001 April; 24(4):351–6.
17. **A** Fries JF. Aging natural death and compression of morbidity *N.Engl. J. Med.* 1980 July 17; 303(3):130–5.
19. **C** Faddy MJ, et al. Accelerated disappearance of ovarian follicles in midlife. Implications for forecasting menopause. Cellular & Integrative physiology (1992).
20. **D** Maninder Ahuja. Age of menopause and determinants of menopause age: A PAN India survey by IMS. *J Midlife Health.* 2016 Jul-Sep; 7(3): 126–31.
21 **B.** Morito K, et al. Interaction of phytoestrogens with estrogen receptor X and B. *Biol Pharm bull.* 2001 April; 24(4):351–6.
    I & H Taylor. Immunolocalization of oestrogen receptor β in human tissues. Journal of Molecular endocrinology. 2000;24:145–55. Millas I, et al. Estrogen receptors α and β in non-target organs for hormone action: Review of literature: *Braz J Morphol Sci* 2009 Vol. 26 No. 3–4:193–7.
23. **D** Ellen B. Gold, et al. Factors Related to Age at Natural Menopause: Longitudinal Analyses From *SWAN Am J Epidemiol.* 2013 Jul 1; 178(1): 70–83.
    Purandare CN, Suvarna Khadilkar. Menopause: Current Concepts: Chapter 1. 2004, Jaypee under auspicies of FOGSI.

Demographics

☐ *Suvarna Khadilkar and Meeta*

1. According to the 2011 consensus statement total population of India is:
   A. 1.21 billion
   B. 3 billion
   C. 520.45 million
   D. 2.3 billion

2. According to the 2011 consensus statement what percentage of women contribute to total population of India?
   A. 62%
   B. 70 %
   C. 48.46%
   D. 41%

3. Life expectancy at birth for females in India is projected to be:
   A. 72.3 years
   B. 62 years
   C. 80.4 years
   D. None of the above

4. All are true about projection of population above 50 years in India except:
   A. 10% among current general population of India is above 50 years
   B. Population above 50 is 28% currently
   C. 22% will be above 50 years by 2025
   D. 33% will be above 50 years by 2050

5. Current world population as in 2017 is:
   A. 13 billions
   B. 7.6 billions
   C. 3 billions
   D. None of the above

6. Projected world population in 2050 will be:
   A. 9.6 billions
   B. 6.9 billions
   C. 122 millions
   D. None of the above

7. The estimated mean age of menopause in India is:
   A. 52 years
   B. 45 years
   C. 48 years
   D. 46 years

8. The prevalence of low bone mass is to the extent of:
   A. 62% by the age of 60 years
   B. 80% by the age of 65 years
   C. Both are false
   D. Both are true

9. From the Indian Million Death Study 2009, the major cause of mortality is:
   A. CVD

B. Diabetes

C. Infections

D. Cancer

10. Population studies on projection of burden of cancer at:

    A. Bangalore, Chennai, Delhi and Mumbai showed a statistically significant increase in age adjusted rate over time

    B. Bangalore, Chennai, Delhi and Mumbai showed a statistically significant decrease in age adjusted rate over time

    C. Bangalore, Chennai, Delhi and Mumbai showed no change in age adjusted rate over time

    D. The trends are different at different metros

11. In Bangalore, Chennai, Delhi and Mumbai, cancer cervix has:

    A. Showed a statistically significant decrease in age adjusted incidence rates

    B. The trends are different at different metros

    C. No change in age adjusted rate over time

    D. Showed a statistically significant increase in age adjusted incidence rates

12. In hospital based studies in the age group (15–34 years), breast was the leading cause of cancer except:

    A. Mumbai

    B. Chennai

    C. New Delhi

    D. Bangalore

13. The commonest cancer associated with diabetes and high BMI is:

    A. Breast cancer

    B. Gallbladder

    C. Cervical cancer

    D. None of the above

Answer Key

1. A	4. B	7. D	10. A	13. A
2. C	5. B	8. D	11. A	
3. A	6. A	9. A	12. D	

References

1. **A** Statistics Division, Ministry of Health and Family Welfare, Government of India. Family Welfare Statistics in India. National Rural Health Mission. 2011.

2. **C** Mithal A, *et al. Indian Journal of Endocrinology and Metabolism.* 2014; 18(4):449–54.

3. **A** Meeta, Digumarti L, Agarwal N, Vaze N, Shah R, Malik S. Clinical practice guidelines on menopause: *An executive summary and recommendations. J Midlife Health* 2013; 4:77–106.

4. **B** Three-Year Report of the PBCRs: 2012–2014 Trends over time and projection of burden of cancer consolidated report of the HBCRs: 2012–2014.

5. **B** Diabetes and adiposity cause 1 in 20 cancers worldwide medscape Nov 29, 2017 https://www.medscape.com/viewarticle/889302

Hormones at Menopause and Hypothalamo-Pituitary-Ovarian Axis

▣ *Navneet Takkar*

1. Anti mullerian hormone (AMH) a marker of ovarian reserve is produced by:
   A. Granulosa cells
   B. Germinal epithelium
   C. Cumulus oophorus
   D. Gonadal-ridge epithelial like cell

2. Hormone changes prior to menopause (perimenopause) is marked by:
   A. Elevated FSH, increased levels of inhibin and normal levels of LH
   B. Elevated FSH, increased levels of inhibin and elevated levels of LH
   C. Elevated FSH, decreased levels of inhibin and normal levels of LH
   D. Normal FSH, decreased levels of inhibin and normal levels of LH

3. Circulating level of estrone in post-menopausal women is:
   A. 10–20 pg/ml
   B. 30–70 pg/ml
   C. 50–80 pg/ml
   D. 80–100 pg/ml

4. The change in androgen/estrogen ratio in menopause is reflected by:
   A. Decline in both androgen and estrogen in equal amounts
   B. Decline in estrogen but slight rise in androgen
   C. Marked decline in estrogen relative to androgen

5. Most of the postmenopausal androstenedione is derived from:
   A. Ovary
   B. Adipose tissue
   C. Adrenal gland
   D. Kidney

6. In menopausal women, FSH levels are higher than LH because:
   A. LH is cleared from the blood faster
   B. LH is production is less as compared to FSH production
   C. Ageing of pituitary gonadotro-pin secreting cells with decreased ability to respond to GnRH

7. Shortly after menopause the androgens secreted by the ovary are:
   A. DHEA and DHEAS
   B. DHEA and androstenedione
   C. DHEA and testosterone
   D. Androstenedione and testosterone

8. Which of the following factors are associated with later onset of menopause:
   A. Smoking and prior use of contraceptives

B. Increased BMI and high altitude living
C. Type I diabetes mellitus and stress
D. Increased BMI and multiparty

9. As per the result of the SWAN study, association between changes in oestradiol and FSH levels during menopausal transition and risk of diabetes:
   A. Lower premenopausal oestradiol levels and a slower rate of FSH level change were associated with higher risk of diabetes
   B. Higher premenopausal oestradiol levels and higher rate of FSH level change were associated with higher risk of diabetes
   C. Higher premenopausal oestradiol and slower rate of FSH level changes were associated with higher risk of diabetes
   D. Lower premenopausal oestradiol changes were associated with higher risk of diabetes

10. Important negative feedback regulations of circulating FSH are:
    A. AMH and iinhibin
    B. Oestradiol and inhibin
    C. Progesterone
    D. AMH and oestradiol

11. Patients suspected of Alzheimer's disease (AD) all the following investigations will aid diagnosis, except:
    A. Thyroid function test
    B. Vitamin B_{12} level
    C. Serum electrolytes

D. Biomarkers like β or tau protein in CSF

12. The predominant oestrogen at menopause is:
    A. Estrone
    B. Estradiol
    C. Estriol

13. Million women study designed to examine different HRT regimens was conducted in:
    A. USA
    B. UK
    C. France
    D. South America

14. Natural estrogens are:
    A. C 17 compound
    B. C 18 compound
    C. C 19 compound
    D. C 21 compound

15. Unopposed oestrogen in women with natural menopause is associated with:
    A. Increased risk of lung cancer
    B. Increased risk of endometrial cancer
    C. Increased risk of colorectal cancer
    D. Increased risk of ovarian cancer

16. Androgens are:
    A. C 17 compound
    B. C 18 compound
    C. C 19 compound
    D. C 21 compound

17. Progesterone are:
    A. C 17 compound
    B. C 18 compound
    C. C 19 compound
    D. C 21 compound

Answer Key

1. A	4. C	7. D	10. B	13. B	16. C
2. C	5. C	8. D	11. C	14. B	17. D
3. B	6. A	9. A	12. A	15. B	

Reference

Purandare CN, Suvarna Khadilkar, Menopause: Current Concepts: 2004, Jaypee under auspicies of FOGSI.

Chapter 4

Effect of Menopause on Body Tissues

◙ *Navneet Takkar*

1. Older skin is predominantly adversely affected by all the following factors except:
    A. Chronological aging
    B. Vitamin E therapy
    C. Estrogen deficiency
    D. Photoaging

2. All of the following skin changes are in sequence to menopause except:
    A. Hyperpigmentation
    B. Increase in sebaceous gland secration
    C. Loss of elasticity
    D. Diminished blood supply

3. The strongest predictor of coronary heart disease in a woman is:
    A. ↑LDL cholesterol
    B. ↓VLDL cholesterol
    C. ↓CRP levels
    D. ↓HDL cholesterol

4. Possible explanation for dry eye syndrome of menopause is:
    A. Lack of estrogen
    B. Fall of systemic androgen levels
    C. Erratic levels of estrogen
    D. None of the above

5. Osteoporosis is a skeletal disease characterized by:
    A. Deterioration of microarchitecture of bone
    B. Low bone mass
    C. Increased bone fragility
    D. All of the above

6. Osteoporosis is also called:
    A. Silent epidemic
    B. Osteopesia
    C. Osteogesia
    D. All of above

7. Bone loss per year in postmenopausal osteoporosis (rapid loosers Type 1) is:
    A. 1.6%
    B. 1.2%
    C. 6.0%
    D. 3.5%

8. The Potential for primary prevention of Alzheimer's disease by estrogen therapy is applicable in which stage of menopause?
    A. Very early in the post menopause
    B. After 5 years
    C. After 10 years
    D. After 20 years

9. Stage +2 as per STRAW classification denotes:
    A. Early reproductive period
    B. Early menopausal transition
    C. Late postmenopause
    D. Late reproductive period

10. ELITE (early versus late intervention trial with estradiol) study was done to know:
    A. Association of vasomotor symptoms and MHT
    B. Osteoporosis and MHT use
    C. Cardiovascular health and MHT use
    D. Sexual health and MHT use

11. Women experiencing vasomotor symptoms should never be prescribed:
    A. Tibolone
    B. Estrogen + progesterone (MHT)
    C. Raloxifene
    D. All of the above

12. A woman with known hypertension requires HT for vasomotor symptoms. The best progesterone in the HT regimen would be:
    A. Natural micronized progesterone
    B. Dydrogesterone
    C. Medroxyprogesteroneacetate
    D. Drosperinone

13. WHI memory study showed:
    A. Decreased risk of dementia in women older than 65 years and HT use
    B. No significant relation between dementia and HT use
    C. Increased risk of dementia in women older than 65 years and HT use
    D. None of the above

14. Hormone therapy in menopausal women protects against all except:
    A. Osteoporosis
    B. Dyspareunia
    C. Stroke
    D. Vaginal atrophy

15. After menopause, the risk of developing cardiovascular disease is increased by:
    A. 5-fold higher risk
    B. 2-fold higher risk
    C. 7-fold higher risk
    D. None of the above

16. As per the results of WISE (women's ischemia syndrome evaluation) heart disease in women is often under diagnosed because:
    A. Atherosclerotic plaque in women is more fibrotic and less vulnerable for plaque rupture
    B. Diffuse atherosclerotic of large vessels is a major cause of ischemia
    C. Women present with acute ischemia syndrome rather than unstable angina
    D. Vascular dysfunction affects smaller vessels that supply the heart and does not show-up on an angiogram

17. Which of the following is recommended currently for prevention of coronary artery disease?
    A. Menopausal hormone therapy
    B. Lifestyle interventions
    C. Aspirin therapy
    D. Use of antioxidant supplements

18. The Framingham risk score, the major risk factors for CVD are all except:
    A. Cigarette smoking
    B. High HDL
    C. Family history of premature CHD
    D. Hypertension

19. State true or false: 'Routine use of aspirin in women is not recommended for myocardial infarction prevention':
    A. True   B. False

20. As per the, The National Cholesterol Education Program, Adult Treatment Plan III, optimal levels of lipids in Indian women:
    A. LDL > 100 mg/dl HDL > 50 mg/dl and TG < 150 mg/dl
    B. LDL < 100 mg/dl HDL < 50 mg/dl and TG < 150 mg/dl
    C. LDL < 100 mg/dl HDL > 50 mg/dl and TG < 150 mg/dl
    D. LDL < 100 mg/dl HDL < 50 mg/dl and TG > 150 mg/dl

21. State true or false 'Incidence of venous thrombo embolism (VTE) is increased in postmenopausal women':
    A. True
    B. False

22. Among all osteoporotic fractures which is the most serious:
    A. Hip fracture
    B. Vertebral fractures
    C. Fracture of forearm
    D. Rib fracture

23. Risk factors for sarcopenia include all except:
    A. Menopausal status
    B. Low physical activity
    C. Low protein intake
    D. Sleep disorders

24. Which of the following is NOT a criteria as per the standardized definition of sarcopenia described by Fried, et al?
    A. Unintentional weight loss
    B. Self-reported exhaustion
    C. Fragility fracture
    D. Slow motor performance

25. All of the following are used in the management of overactive bladder (OAB) in menopausal women except:
    A. Burch colpo suspension
    B. Bladder drill
    C. Oxybutynin
    D. Kegel exercises

26. Female sexual dysfunction includes all of following sexual disorders except:
    A. Hypoactive sexual desire dis-order
    B. Vaginismus
    C. Vulvodynia
    D. Dyspareunia

27. As per the SWAN (study of women's health across the nation) which of the following factor is protective for hot flashes:
    A. Obesity
    B. Smoking
    C. Surgical menopause
    D. Caucasian race

28. Which of the following drug is FDA approved non-hormonal management of hot flashes:
    A. Gabapentin
    B. Paroxetine
    C. Clonidine
    D. Lycopene

29. All of the following hair changes are seen in midlife women except:
    A. Hirsutism
    B. Thinning of hair
    C. Hair folliculitis
    D. Androgenic alopecia

30. Ovarian volume goes on decreasing every year after menopause:
    A. $2.6 \pm 2.3 \, cm^3$ in the first menopausal year, to $1.2 \pm 1.4 \, cm^3$ after more than 15 years after the menopause
    B. $8.6 \pm 2.3 \, cm^3$ in the first menopausal year, to $2.2 \pm 1.4 \, cm^3$ after more than 15 years after the menopause
    C. $5.3 \pm 2.3 \, cm^3$ in the first menopausal year, to $3.2 \pm 1.4 \, cm^3$ after more than 15 years after the menopause
    D. None of the above

31. Which is the commonest cause of dementia in ageing women:
    A. Huntington's disease
    B. Multiple sclerosis
    C. Alzheimer's disease
    D. Cerebrovascular disease

32. The heart and estrogen/progestin replacement study (HERS), a clinical trial examining 2763 postmenopausal women with heart disease on ET/EPT versus placebo showed that:
    A. Increase in cardiovascular events in the first year and decrease in events overtime
    B. A significant decrease in the risk of venous thromboembolism (VTE)
    C. An impairment in the lipid profile

D. Decrease in cardiovascular events in first year and increase in events overtime

33. The PEPI trial (postmenopausal estrogen-progestin intervention trial) showed that:
    A. A substantial increase in LDL cholesterol in women on EPT
    B. No effect on lipid metabolism in women on estrogen-progestin therapy
    C. Micronized progesterone did not adversely affect the beneficial effects on lipids of estrogens
    D. None of the above

34. The rate of bone loss during early menopause is usually:
    A. 0.3 to 0.5% per year
    B. 4 to 5% per year
    C. 8 to 10% per year
    D. 2 to 3% per year

35. Effects of menopause on bone metabolism include all except:
    A. Acceleration of bone loss
    B. Decreased secretion of calcitonin
    C. Decreased calcium absorption
    D. Increased urinary excretion of calcium and hydroxyproline
    E. Increased osteoblastic activity

36. Hand-held dynamometry is used for diagnosing:
    A. Osteopenia
    B. Nutritional status assessment
    C. Vitamin D deficiency
    D. Sarcopenia

37. The most effective treatment of urogenital atrophy is:
    A. Vaginal estrogen therapy
    B. Vaginal moisturizers
    C. Phytoestrogens
    D. Ospemifene

38. State true or false 'MHT is not a recommended treatment for meno- pausal obstructive sleep apnoea.'
    A. True   **B.** False

39. Treatment of restless leg syndrome includes all except:
    A. Avoidance of alcohol and caffe- ine
    B. Avoidance of antidepressants
    C. Lithium therapy
    D. Replace iron if iron level is low

40. The most important treatment to improve the muscle mass used in treatment of sarcopenia is:
    A. Acupuncture
    B. Vitamin D and calcium supplemen- tation
    C. Progressive resistance training
    D. Myostatin therapy

41. Vaginal atrophy becomes clinically apparent in:
    A. Perimenopause
    B. 8–10 years after menopause
    C. At the time menopause
    D. 2–3 years after menopause

42. The drug which is FDA approved for treatment of moderate to severe dyspareunia is:
    A. Tibolone
    B. Ospemifene
    C. Dehydroepiandrosterone (DHEA)
    D. Genistein

43. All are early menopausal effects except:
    A. Psychological disturbances
    B. Hot flushes
    C. Osteoporosis
    D. Sleep disturbance

44. Maximum bone density and strength is reached around the age:
    A. 30 years
    B. 20 years
    C. 25 years
    D. 45 years

45. All of the following are causes of secondary osteoporosis except:
    A. Amyloidosis
    B. Multiple myeloma
    C. Increasing age
    D. Chronic kidney disease

46. State true or false 'As per the Rancho Bernado study, women who used MHT continuously or intermittently over a 15-year follow-up had significantly higher BMI, than women who never used it.'
    A. True
    B. False

47. Estrogen leads to following effect on levels of high density lipoprotein (HDL):
    A. Decrease
    B. Increase
    C. Remain the same
    D. Effect is variable

48. HERS (heart estrogen-progesterone replacement study) ended after 4.1 years due to:
    A. It proved efficiency of estrogen as cardioprotective agent
    B. It showed no change in lipid profile of estrogen user
    C. Coronary events increased by 50% during the first year of trial
    D. All of the above

49. The largest study of WHI (womens health initiative) of estrogen+progesterone therapy, following holds true:
    A. It was a randomized study
    B. It was done on 16,608 subjects
    C. It was halted prematurely in July 2002
    D. All of the above

50. WHI project halted prematurely in 2002 instead of 2005 due to all of the following reasons except:
    A. Increased rate of coronary events in HRT users
    B. Increased incidence of stroke in HRT users
    C. Administration and financial problems
    D. Two-fold rise in the risk of venous thromboembolism

51. Neuroendocrine changes in menopausal age group are implicated for:
    A. Hot flushes and night sweats
    B. Sleep disturbances
    C. Mood disturbances
    D. Memory and cognition
    E. All of the above

52. Pick out the false statement:
    A. Estrogen has a neuroprotective role
    B. A temporal correlation exist between occurrence of hot flushes and LH-LHRH
    C. Declining estrogen levels at menopause seem to be the common neuroendocrine mechanism for insomnia and hot flushes
    D. 'Menopausal Blues' have more prevalence of symptoms in women from eastern countries than the western counterparts

53. The main metabolite of brain norepinephrine, implicated before hot flushes:
    A. MHPG (3 methoxy–4 hydroxy-phenylglycol)
    B. POMC (pro-opiomelanocortin)
    C. Opioids
    D. Tachykinins

54. In symptomatic women with hot flushes the following would pro-voke hot flushes:
    A. Yohimbine (α 2 adrenergic antagonist)
    B. Clonidine (α 2 adrenergic agonist)
    C. Reserpine
    D. All of the above

55. True of false:
    A. Estrogen levels correlate well with hot flushes
    B. Estrogen replacement during menopausal transition virtually eliminates vasomotor symptoms
    C. Considerable evidence exists for estrogen modulation of central nor-adrenergic activity

D. Trials show that maximum benefit of MHT for sleep restoration is observed in women with coexistent hot flushes

56. Pick out the correct statement about neuroprotective role of estrogen:
   A. In clinical practice as opposed to experimental animal models, estrogen is neuroprotective
   B. Estrogen therapy beyond 10 years of menopause has a neuroprotective role in Alzhiemer's
   C. Experimental data suggest neuroprotective role of estrogen and clinical studies do not support it
   D. All of the above

Answer Key

1. B	11. C	21. B	31. C	41. B	51. E
2. B	12. D	22. A	32. A	42. B	52. D
3. D	13. C	23. D	33. C	43. C	53. A
4. B	14. C	24. C	34. D	44. A	54. A
5. D	15. B	25. A	35. E	45. C	55. A False
6. A	16. D	26. C	36. D	46. B	B, C, D
7. C	17. B	27. A	37. A	47. B	True
8. A	18. B	28. B	38. A	48. C	56. C
9. C	19. A	29. C	39. C	49. D	
10. C	20. C	30. B	40. C	50. C	

References and Explanations

8. **A.** Studies have shown early use of estrogen reduces incidence of Alzheimer's, and late use worsens Alzheimer Henderson VW, Benke KS, Green RC, Cupples LA, Farrer LA. Postmenopausal hormone therapy and Alzheimer's disease risk: interaction with age. *Journal of Neurology, Neurosurgery,* and *Psychiatry.* 2005;76:103–5.

17. **B.** MHT is not recommended for primary, secodary or tertiary prevention of cardiac protection whereas lifestyle changes are recommended aspirin may be indicated only in high-risk groups and antioxidants supplements are not recommended.

19. **A.** Women who are at high cardiometabbolic risk women are given aspirin and not all women routinely.

28. Clonidine used commonly but is off label so only paroxetine is FDA approved.

Types of Menopause, Risks and Management

◼ *Seema Sharma and Preeti Deshpande*

1. All of the following are characteristic features of primary ovarian in sufficiency except:
   A. Amenorrhoea
   B. Hypoestrogenism
   C. Elevated *S. gonadotrophins*
   D. ↑ACTH

2. Which of the following is correct in relation to women with premature ovarian failure?
   A. Women with POF are not at increased risk of osteoporosis-related fracture
   B. They should encourage to take HRT for a total duration of 5 years and stop it after 5 years
   C. HRT suppresses spontaneous ovulation and will provide an effective contraception
   D. The combined contraceptive pill can be used as an alternative to HRT for control of menopausal symptoms and protection against osteoporosis and CVS disease

3. Premature ovarian failure may be due to following reason:
   A. Toxic exposure
   B. Autoimmune disorder
   C. Chromosomal abnormality
   D. All of the above

4. In surgically induced menopause, following are true except:
   A. Symptoms start instantaneously
   B. Affects > 90% of patients
   C. Early use of ET alleviates symptoms
   D. Testosterone is not needed

5. Surgical menopause may be accompanied by cognitive impairment that primarily affects verbal episodic memory while natural menopause is not accompanied by substantial changes in cognitive abilities.
   A. True
   B. False

6. Which of the following single gene perturbations predispose to premature ovarian insufficiency-
   A. BMP 15 538 A
   B. C-RAS
   C. Her 2 neu
   D. HE4

7. Which of the following gene perturbation is found associated with premature ovarian insufficiency:
   A. FMR1 Xq27.3 (oocyte development and maturation)
   B. Inhibin α 769 (INHA 769)
   C. GDF – 95q23.2 (follicular maturation)

D. Newborn ovary Homobox gene [NOBOX 7q25](early folliculogenesis)

E. All of the above

8. All of the following gene perturbations are associated with premature ovarian insufficiency except:
   A. ER and gene polymorphism
   B. FMR – 1 permutation on X chromosome
   C. INHA 769
   D. PGRMC – 1

9. Which of the following studies are currently being used to reveal loci not predicted by candidate genes for studying gene perturbations for premature menopause:
   A. SWAN
   B. MWS
   C. GWAS
   D. NHS

10. Which of the following poly glandular autoimmune diseases can be found in some women with premature ovarian insufficiency:
    A. Autoimmune hypothyroidism
    B. Diabetes mellitus
    C. Adrenal insufficiency
    D. All of the above

11. All of the following are secondary causes of ovarian insufficiency except:
    A. Chemotherapy and radiotherapy
    B. Bilateral oophorectomy
    C. Uterine artery embolization
    D. FMR 1 premutations

12. All of the following are primary causes of premature ovarian insufficiency except:
    A. Chromosome abnormalities
    B. Uterine artery embolization
    C. Enzyme deficiencies
    D. Autoimmune diseases

13. Diagnostic usefulness of which of the following investigation is not proven for routine use to investigate the cases of premature ovarian insufficiency:
    A. AMH
    B. Inhibin – B
    C. Ovarian biopsy
    D. Chromosomal analysis for women younger than 30 years

14. Which of the following investigations are indicated in cases of premature ovarian insufficiency:
    A. Hormone analysis including: FSH, LH, estradiol, AMH, inhibin–B, prolactin
    B. Autoimmune screen for poly endocrinopathies
    C. Pelvic and breast ultrasound
    D. All of the above
    E. None of the above

15. Which of the following is only an optional investigation in patients with premature ovarian insufficiency:
    A. Screen for autoimmune polyendocrinopathies
    B. Pelvic and breast ultrasound
    C. Dual X-ray absorptiometry
    D. Chromosome analysis for women younger than 30 years

16. All of the following are true for therapeutic options of premature ovarian insufficiency except:
    A. They need higher doses of estrogens compared to women over 40 years old.
    B. The aim is to achieve the typical mean serum estradiol levels of approximately 400 mg/ml.
    C. Recommended estrogen doses are 17 β estradiol 2 mg/ml or 1.25 mg conjugated quine estrogen or transdermal estradiol 75–100 µg/day or µgm ethinylestradiol.
    D. Micronized progesterone can be administered as cyclic regimen or as a continuous regimen of 100 mg per day.

17. According to reproductive endocrinology special interest group of ESHRE guideline on premature ovarian insufficiency definition of POI includes all expect:
    A. Loss of ovarian activity before the age of 40
    B. Menstrual disturbance
    C. Raised gonadotropins
    D. Low estradiol
    E. High AMH

18. Prevalence of premature ovarian insufficiency is approximately:
    A. 1%
    B. 9%
    C. 11%
    D. 19%

19. In view of the long-term health consequence of POI effort should be made to modify the following factors:
    A. Gynaecological surgical practice
    B. Lifestyle factor
    C. Modified treatment regimens for malignant and chronic disease
    D. All of the above
    E. None of the above

20. Considering the history primary ovarian insufficiency was first described in
    A. 1742
    B. 1842
    C. 1942
    D. 1642

21. A 32-year-old female presented with hyper pigmentation, recurrent candidiasis, amenorrhoea since one year. Her TSH found to be 62 IU/ml and anti TPO antibody level 23. Her FSH on 2 different Occasions 4 Weeks apart was >25 IU/L. On genetic testing AIRE mutation was present. Most appropriate diagnosis for her is:
    A. DiGeorge syndrome
    B. WDHA syndrome
    C. Autoimmune polyglandular syndrome 2 (APS–2)
    D. Autoimmune polyglandular syndrome–1 (APS–1)

22. Premature menopause occurs before the age of:
    A. 40 years
    B. 35 years
    C. 42 years
    D. 45 years

23. Menopause is referred to as 'Late menopause' if it occurs after the age of:
    A. 50 years
    B. 51 years
    C. 52 years
    D. 55 years

24. Surgical menopause occurs due to:
    A. Bilateral oophorectomy
    B. Hysterectomy
    C. Chemoablation
    D. Hysterectomy and bilateral oophorectomy
    E. (A) and (D) are correct
    F. (A), (B) and (D) are correct

25. What is chemical menopause?
    A. Induced by a drug for short-term
    B. Chemotherapy
    C. Radiation
    D. All of the above

26. Potential beneficial effect of surgical menopause is maximum in:
    A. Woman with risk of cancer ovary
    B. Pelvic pain in endometriosis
    C. None of these
    D. (A) and (B) are correct

27. Risk of surgical menopause is:
    A. Severe menopausal symptoms like hot flushes
    B. Reduced bone mineral density
    C. Reduced sex drive
    D. Loss of fertility
    E. Cardiovascular risk
    F. All of the above

28. Premature ovarian failure is the same as:
    A. Premature menopause

B. Primary ovarian insufficiency
C. Both of the above
D. None of the above

29. Premature ovarian failure is the loss of normal function of ovaries before the age of:
    A. 40 years
    B. 35 years
    C. 30 years
    D. 20 years

30. Women with premature ovarian failure:
    A. Can have irregular periods for years and can get pregnant
    B. Cannot get pregnant
    C. Can have complete cessation of period
    D. Can get pregnant

31. Causes of premature ovarian failure are:
    A. Chromosomal defect
    B. Toxins like chemotherapy/ radio-therapy
    C. Autoimmune conditions
    D. Idiopathic factors
    E. Multiple ovarian surgery
    F. All of the above

32. Incidence of premature ovarian failure is:
    A. 0.5–3%
    B. 5–10%
    C. > 10%
    D. Unknown

33. Complication of premature ovarian failure:
    A. Infertility
    B. Osteoporosis
    C. Depression/anxiety
    D. Heart disease
    E. Dementia
    F. All of the above

34. Early menopause increases risk of osteoporotic fractures as compared to normal menopause by:
    A. Double

B. Triple
C. Quadruple
D. Slightly

35. Early menopause occurs:
    A. Before 40 years of age
    B. At 41–45 years age
    C. At 45–49 years age
    D. At 42 years of age

36. Premature menopause is associated with:
    A. Long-term negative effect on cognitive function
    B. Dementia
    C. Both of the above
    D. None of the above

37. Familial premature ovarian failure can occur due to:
    A. Partial deletion of the long arm of X chromosome (Xq)
    B. Partial deletion of the short arm of X chromosome (Xp)
    C. Both of the above
    D. Unknown genetic defect

38. Late menopause is associated with
    A. Diabetes type 2
    B. HT
    C. Hypothyroidism
    D. None of the above

39. Late age at menopause has been associated with:
    A. Increased risk of cardiovascular disease
    B. Stroke
    C. Angina
    D. Breast/endometrial and ovarian cancer

40. The following lifestyle/dietary factors delay onset of menopause:
    A. Smoking
    B. Alcohol
    C. Green/yellow vegetables rich in carotene
    D. Meat/non-vegetarian food

41. Early menopause protects against:
    A. Osteoporosis

B. Urine infection
C. Breast cancer
D. Ovarian cancer

42. Age of menopause is influenced by:
    A. Genetics
    B. Socioeconomic status
    C. Dietary habits
    D. All of the above

43. In the following conditions higher dose of hormone therapy is required
    A. Natural menopause
    B. Surgical menopause
    C. Premature menopause
    D. Both (B) and (C)
    E. None of the above

Answer Key

1. D	9. C	17. E	25. A	33. F	41. C
2. D	10. D	18. A	26. D	34. A	42. D
3. D	11. D	19. D	27. F	35. B	43. D
4. D	12. C	20. C	28. B	36. A	
5. A	13. C	21. D	29. A	37. A	
6. A	14. D	22. A	30. A	38. A	
7. E	15. C	23. D	31. F	39. D	
8. A	16. B	24. E	32. A	40. C	

Explanation

9.   **C**   Studies performed in Serbian women showed that estrogen receptor and gene polymorphism is not associated with POI.

10. **D**   Whole genome approaches, e.g. Genome Wide Association Studies (GWAS), are being used to reveal loci not predicted by candidate genes. Karyotype methodology has detected monosomy X, mosaicism, X chromosome deletions and rearrangements, X autosome translocations, and isochromosomes in women with POI.

12. **C**   Fragile–X–mental retardation 1 premutation on X-chromosome are primary causes of POI rest all are secondary causes.

14. **D**   The diagnostic usefulness of ovarian biopsy outside the context of a research setting is unproven.

17. **E**   The aim is to achieve the typical mean serum estradiol levels of approximately 100 pg/ml (400 pmol) lt in regularly menstruating women.

18. **A**   AMH is not included in ESHRE definition

22. **A**   Autoimmune Polyglandular Syndrome–1 is a rare autosomal recessive disease caused by mutation in the AIRE gene mainly presenting as candidiasis hypoparathyroidism and Addison's disease, ovarian insufficiency occurs in 15% of cases.

40. **C**   41. **C**, 42. **D**: https://www.healthline.com/health/menopause/menopause-age Ahuja M. Age of menopause and determinants of menopause age: A PAN India survey by IMS. J Mid-life Health 2016; 7:126–31.

Clinical Symptoms and Signs of Menopause

◉ *Seema Sharma*

1. During SWAN study information was collected from 3, 302 midlife women annually regarding:
   A. Vasomotor and other menopause related symptoms
   B. Health behaviour
   C. Social and psychological functioning
   D. Physiologic indices
   E. All of the above
   F. None of the above

2. Under SWAN study the participants– (3, 302 midlife women across 5 racial/ ethnic groups) are in which year of their follow-up in 2017:
   A. 2 years
   B. 5 years
   C. 10 years
   D. 23 years

3. All factors are associated with fractures in postmenopausal women except:
   A. Increasing age
   B. Low body weight (<127 lb / 58 kg)
   C. Family history of osteoporosis
   D. Using hormone therapy

4. All are true regarding bacterial vaginosis except:
   A. Most common infections as vaginal pH and flora is altered due to loss of estrogen
   B. More common with multiple sex partners and new sex partners, also with women having IUCD
   C. May be asymptomatic or just have fishy odor discharge
   D. Vaginal pH/KOH (with test)/ clue cell test needed to confirm
   E. Treatment of the condition is not mandatory

5. Investigation of premature menopause; which test is optional?
   A. Estimates of levels of follicle-stimulating hormone in serum
   B. Thyroid function tests
   C. Chromosome analysis, especially in women younger than 30 years
   D. Estimates of bone mineral density through dual X-ray absorptiometry (DEXA)

6. Which is the most common cause of postmenopausal bleeding?
   A. Endometrial atrophy
   B. Endometrial hyperplasia
   C. Endometrial polyp
   D. Cancer endometrium

7. Which of the following statement is most suitable for vasomotor symptoms after menopause?
   A. Placebo is as effective as MHT in managing vasomotor symptoms
   B. Treatment should be restricted to a maximum duration of 5 years
   C. Women should be encouraged to stop MHT by the age of 60 years.
   D. Vasomotor symptom is the most common indication for prescribing MHT.

8. How are hot flushes normally described?
   A. A sudden feeling of heat to the trunk and face that quickly spreads to the rest of the body. The duration is between seconds to 2–3 minutes
   B. Sudden feeling of heat to the trunk and face that quickly spreads to the rest of the body. The duration is between minutes to a couple of hours
   C. Sudden feeling of heat to the arms and legs. The duration is between seconds to 2–3 minutes
   D. A generalized feeling of heat to all body, accompanied by palpitation and anxiety

9. Perimenopausal sleep disturbances are said to be significant when their frequency:
   A. Once in a month for 6 months
   B. Once in a week for 2 months
   C. At least 3 nights per week for a month
   D. None of the above

10. A 55-year-old woman with her final menstrual period at age 50, presents with h/o light vaginal bleeding for 3 days you should:
   A. Give her vaginal estrogen for atrophic vaginitis and tell her to come if bleeding does not stop
   B. Perform TAH with BSO to R/o CA endometrium
   C. Take history, perform physical examination, perform endometrial biopsy/USS/hysteroscopy

11. Trials show that maximum benefit of MHT for sleep restoration is observed in women with co-existent hot flushes.
   A. True
   B. False

12. Estrogen replacement during menopausal transition virtually eliminates vasomotor symptoms.
   A. True
   B. False

13. Estrogen levels correlate well with hot flushes.
   A. True
   B. False

14. Following postmenopausal symptoms occur due to estrogen lack:
   A. Urinary incontinence
   B. Genital prolapse
   C. Dyspareunia
   D. All of the above

15. Menorrhagia is a common perimenopausal symptoms:
   A. True
   B. False
   C. Cannot say
   D. None of the above

16. Differential diagnosis of hot flushes are:
   A. Pheochromocytoma
   B. Thyroid disease
   C. None of the two
   D. Both A and B

17. Which of the following is not true about postmenopausal hot flush?
   A. Coincides with the surge of LH
   B. There is a subjective prodromal awareness of beginning of flush
   C. Prodrome is followed by measurable increased heat over the entire body surface
   D. Does not occur after hypophysectomy

18. In Massachusetts women's health study the incidence of hot flushes was maximum during:
    A. Premenopausal period
    B. Just after cessation of menses
    C. Late postmenopausal period
    D. No effect of menopause status

19. All of the following are risk factors for hot flushes except:
    A. Surgical menopause
    B. Smoking
    C. White races
    D. High circulating levels of estradiol

20. Systolic blood pressure increased during an episode of hot flush occurring of either during sleep or while being awake state true or false:
    A. True
    B. False

21. In the postmenopausal estrogen progestin interventions (PEPI) trial the percentage of women 55–64 years old who were sexually active was:
    A. 40%
    B. 60%
    C. 80%
    D. 85%

22. Which of the following is not the classical symptom of menopause:
    A. Hot flushes
    B. Sweating
    C. Excessive sleep
    D. Vaginal dryness

23. According to wise study—Severe vasomotor symptoms have been linked to all of the following except:
    A. Increased intima media thickness
    B. Aortic calcification
    C. Increased brachial artery flow – mediated dilation (FMD)
    D. Adverse CVD risk factors 8–10

24. Which of the following statements about menopausal hot flashes is TRUE?
    A. About 25% of menopausal women experience hot flashes
    B. Hot flashes most frequently subside 2 years after menopause
    C. Women can continue to experience hot flashes for 10 years after menopause
    D. Smokers are less likely to experience hot flashes than nonsmokers

25. Women in the WHI who were treated with combined estrogen-progesterone therapy had a lower risk of experiencing which of the following outcomes compared to the placebo group?
    A. Breast cancer
    B. Stroke
    C. CHD
    D. Colon cancer

26. Mrs X is a non-smoker and her only medical problem is hypertension, which is well-controlled with hydrochlorothiazide. She has never had any abnormal mammograms, breast biopsies, or gynecologic surgeries. Her mother had a heart attack at the age of 65. What do you tell Mrs X about her risk for MI with combination E+P therapy?
    A. She should avoid combination E+P therapy altogether, because it will substantially increase her risk for MI
    B. E+P therapy will increase her risk for MI now, but if she waits until she is 62 she can safely start it
    C. She should wait to start E+P therapy until she is later in menopause, because it seems to be safer then
    D. She should start E+P therapy now, as her baseline risk for MI is low

27. All of the following have been shown to be effective for reducing hot flashes except:
    A. Placebo
    B. Wellbutrin

C. Gabapentin

D. Venlafaxine

28. What herbal therapies have been shown to be effective for treating menopausal hot flashes?

A. Phytoestrogens

B. Black cohosh

C. Red clover

D. All of the above

29. Mrs X 49 years old, suffering from severe vaginal dryness. She gives family history of MI to mother at 65 years of age and recently diagnosed breast cancer to her sister. All of the following would be effective treatment regimens for except.

A. 10 mcg intravaginal estrogen ring (replaced every 3 months)

B. Intravaginal 25 mcg estrogen tablet, used daily for 2 weeks and then twice per week

C. Vaginal moisturizer applied daily every 3 days

D. Vaginal lubricant applied prior to intercourse

30. Women who are going through menopause should take:

A. Hormone therapy

B. Estrogen therapy

C. Bioidentical hormone therapy

D. Tailored therapy based on symptoms and medical history

31. The most accurate test to determine if a woman is perimenopausal is:

A. Follicle stimulating hormone (FSH) blood levels

B. Complete blood count

C. S. Progesterone levels

D. None of the above

32. The main metabolite of brain norepinephrine, implicated for hot flushes:

A. MHPG (3 methoxy – 4 hydroxy-phenylgycol)

B. POMC (Pro-opiomelanocortin)

C. Opioids

D. Tachykinins

33. In symptomatic women with hot flushes, following would provoke hot flushes:

A. Yohimbine (α 2 adrenergic antagonist)

B. Clonidine (α 2 adrenergic agonist)

C. Reserpine

D. All of the above

34. Regarding estrogen and CAD all are true except:

A. In the presence of atherosclerosis estrogen may not be able to increase the activity of nitric oxide

B. Estrogens though have beneficial effects over lipids, yet short-term improvement in lipids are not able to affect coronary lesions when they are extensive

C. Transdermal estrogen is not preferred in high-risk patients having metabolic syndrome with enhanced CVS risk

D. Oral administration of estrogen increases C-reactive proteins and it may be hazardous in women with CAD

35. More common presentations of CAD in women are:

A. Women presenting at later age than men

B. In women, typical symptoms of angina are less common presentation of CAD

C. Women may present with shoulder or jaw pain, dyspnoea or nausea

D. Suffocating type of chest pain with sweating and dyspnoea

E. All of the above

36. All of the following are risk factors for Alzheimer's disease except:

A. Advancing age

B. Genetic

C. Diabetes

D. High level of physical activity

37. The following laboratory findings are associated with atrophic vaginitis except:

A. S. FSH > 40 IU/ml

B. S. Estrogen < 29 pg/ml

C. Low vaginal PH < 4

D. Thin endometrium of TVS <5 mm.

38. Menorrhagia is the commonest perimenopausal symptom.

A. True

B. False

39. In perimenopause which type of incontinence is more frequent:

A. Urge incontinence

B. True incontinence

C. Stress incontinence

D. All of the above

40. Women experiencing perimenopausal symptoms should never be prescribed:

A. Estrogen: Progesterone

B. Tibolone

C. Raloxifene

D. All of the above

Answer Key

1. E	8. A	15. B	22. C	29. D	36. D
2. D	9. C	16. D	23. C	30. D	37. C
3. D	10. C	17. D	24. C	31. D	38. B
4. E	11. A	18. B	25. D	32. A	39. C
5. D	12. A	19. D	26. D	33. A	40. C
6. A	13. B	20. A	27. B	34. C	
7. D	14. D	21. B	28. D	35. E	

Explanations

Answer 1 and 2: http://www.swanstudy.org/

The Study of Women's Health Across the Nation (SWAN) is a multi-site longitudinal, epidemiologic study designed to examine the health of women during their middle years. The study examines the physical, biological, psychological and social changes during this transitional period. The goal of SWAN's research is to help scientists, health care providers and women learn how midlife experiences affect health and quality of life during aging. The study is co-sponsored by the National Institute on Aging (NIA), the National Institute of Nursing Research (NINR), the National Institutes of Health (NIH), Office of Research on Women's Health, and the National Center for Complementary and Alternative Medicine.

The study began in 1994 and is in its twenty-second year. Between 1996 and 1997, 3,302 participants joined SWAN through seven designated research centers. The research centers are located in the following communities: Ann Arbor, MI (University of Michigan), Boston, MA (Massachusetts General Hospital), Chicago, IL (Rush University Medical Center), Alameda and Contra Costa County, CA (University of California Davis and Kaiser Permanente), Los Angeles, CA (University of California at Los Angeles), Jersey City, NJ (Albert Einstein College of Medicine), and Pittsburgh, PA (University of Pittsburgh). SWAN participants represent five racial/ethnic groups and a variety of backgrounds and cultures.

23.   **C** More frequent or severe VMS have been linked to adverse CVD risk factors 8–10 and subclinical CVD, such as Increased intima media thickness, aortic calcification reduced brachial artery flow mediated dilation (FMD) – a marker of endothelial dysfunction. Women's ischemia syndrome evaluation (WISE).

Investigation at and around Menopause

■ *Ambuja*

1. The cut-off value of measurement of endometrial thickness in postmeno-pausal women with abnormal uterine bleeding above which endo- metrial biopsy is required for evaluation is:
   A. 4 mm
   B. 10 mm
   C. 12 mm
   D. 15 mm

2. Average HDL cholesterol levels in women is approximately:
   A. 55–60 mg/dl
   B. 45–50 mg/dl
   C. 35–40 mg/dl
   D. 25–30 mg/dl

3. In TVS following are associated with endometrial cancer except:
   A. Thick endometrium > 9 mm
   B. Inhomogenous endometrium
   C. Presence of fluid in the cavity
   D. Endometrial thickness < 4 mm

4. 35 years female recently married presented with secondary amenor-rhea of 6 months. Pregnancy test is negative. She has irregular periods and only withdrawal bleeding since 1 year. What test confirms premature ovarian insufficiency (POI)?
   A. Elevated serum gonadotropins
   B. Elevated serum estradiol

C. Elevated inhibin B
D. Atrophic ovries by transvaginal scan

5. One of the feature of overt premature ovarian insufficiency is:
   A. Normal serum gonadotropins
   B. Irregular menses
   C. Normal level of serum estradiol.
   D. Abnormal karyotype

6. Basic hormonal investigation for normal menopausal women:
   A. FSH
   B. AMH
   C. Estradiol
   D. TSH

7. What are not the basic investigations at menopause:
   A. Haemoglobin, plasma glucose, lipid profile
   B. Serum calcium, phosphorus, alkaline phosphatase, 25 hydroxy vitamin D
   C. Dual energy X–ray absorptiometry, mammograpghy
   D. Bone turn over markers

8. What are the indications for DEXA
   A. All postmenopausal women more than 5 years of menopause

B. Postmenopausal women less than 5 years of menopause with risk factors

C. Radiological evidence of osteopenia and presence of vertebral compression fracture

D. Women with fragility fractures

E. All of the above

9. Which of the fallowing are not essential investigations at menopause?
   A. Lipid profile
   B. Serum FSH
   C. Mammography
   D. Ultrasonography

10. 40 years perimenopausal patient routine abdominal ultrasound revealed right sided ovarian cyst of 5 cm diameter. What next?
    A. CA 125
    B. CT scan pelvis
    C. MRI
    D. Transvaginal ultrasound with color Doppler

11. Up to what size of simple ovarian cyst is considered normal physiological in perimenopausal patient?
    A. 3 cm
    B. 5 cm
    C. 7 cm
    D. 8 cm

12. Which of the following is least sensitive method for ovarian cancer screening?
    A. Bimanual pelvic examination
    B. CA 125
    C. Transvaginal sonography
    D. MRI pelvis

13. Routine pelvic examination in a 45 years postmenopausal asymptomatic women revealed adenexal mass of 4 × 5 cm mass best confirmatory test:
    A. X-ray pelvis
    B. CT pelvis
    C. MRI pelvis
    D. 2D ultrasound with Doppler

14. In the same patient USG showed ascitis with extensive disease. Next investigation of choice is:
    A. Fine needle aspiration cytology/biopsy
    B. MRI pelvis
    C. CT pelvis
    D. CA 125

15. Who are the candidates for risk reducing bilateral salpingo oopherectomy?
    A. Early menopause
    B. Late menopause
    C. Women with BRCA mutation
    D. Women with Lynch syndrome

16. Early detection of ovarian cancer is by:
    A. Symptom index
    B. Tumour makers
    C. Ultrasound
    D. MRI

17. What are the significant complaints in symptom complex?
    A. Fever, cachexia, frequency of micturition
    B. Pelvic or abdominal pain
    C. Swelling of lower limbs, constipation, fever
    D. Dyspnoea and palpitation

18. The symptom index is considered to be positive:
    A. If a woman reports any of the below symptoms that are:
       (1) New to her within the past 6 months and
       (2) Occur more than 6 times per month
    B. If a woman reports any of the below symptoms that are:
       (1) New to her within the past 9 months and
       (2) Occur more than 3 times per month
    C. If a woman reports any of the below symptoms that are:
       (1) New to her within the past year and

(2) Occur more than 9 times per month

D. If a woman reports any of the below symptoms that are:
(1) New to her within the past year and
(2) Occur more than 12 times per month

19. Which is not an indication for DEXA?
A. All postmenopausal women more than 5 years of menopause.
B. Postmenopausal women less than 5 years of menopause with risk factors
C. All women in menopause transition.
D. Radiological evidence of osteopenia and presence of vertebral compression fracture

20. Current ATP III criteria to define the metabolic syndrome:
A. Abdominal obesity, defined as a waist circumference in women ≥ 88 cm (35 in)
B. Serum triglycerides ≥ 150 mg/dL (1.7 mmol/L) or drug treatment for elevated triglycerides
C. Serum high-density lipoprotein (HDL) cholesterol < 50 mg/dL (1.3 mmol/L) in women or drug treatment for low HDL cholesterol
D. Blood pressure ≥ 130/85 mmHg or drug treatment for elevated blood pressure
E. Fasting plasma glucose (FPG) ≥ 100 mg/dL (5.6 mmol/L)
F. Presence of any three of the above five traits

21. Breast cancer screening according to ACOG:
A. Clinical breast examination 20 to 39 years every 1 to 3 years—mammaography annually–above 40 years

B. Clinical breast examination 20 to 39 years annually—mammography annually—above 50 years
C. Clinical breast examination–not compulsory–mammography annually—above 50 years
D. Clinical breast examination–not significant—mammography annually 50 to 74 years

22. For dense breast—what is the preferred method for screening?
A. Digital mammography
B. Film mammography
C. Tomosynthesis
D. Ultrasound

23. Investigation to diagnose urogenital syndrome:
A. Urine culture and sensitivity
B. Vaginal pH estimation
C. Pap smear
D. Hysteroscopy

24. The cut-off thickness of endometrium for detection of endometrial disease after 5 years since menopause is:
A. 3 mm
B. 1 mm
C. 2 mm
D. 1.5 mm

25. The correct method of measuring the endometrial thickness by USG is
A. Maximum AP thickness in the sagittal long-axis
B. Maximum AP thickness in the coronal long-axis
C. Maximum AP thickness in the saggital long-axis by excluding the depth of fluid collection
D. Minimum AP thickness in the saggital long-axis

26. Approximately ___ of endometrial cancers occur in postmenopausal women:
A. 50%
B. 60%

C. 70 %

D. 80%

27. As per criteria of texture of endometrium, expectant management in postmenopausal bleeding can be offered to patients with (Sheikh et al 2000):
    A. Homogenous endometrium which is 6 mm thick or less
    B. Heterogenous endometrium which is 6 mm thick or less.
    C. Mixed echogenicity of endometrium
    D. None of the above

28. Ovarian volume in the 1st menopausal year is:
    A. 5+/- 2 ml
    B. 3 ml
    C. 8.6. +/ - 2.3 ml
    D. 4 ml

29. Endometrial atrophy in menopause and appears on the ultrasound as:
    A. Irregular, rugged echogenicity
    B. Pencil-line, echogenicity
    C. Hair-line echogenicity
    D. Mixed thick (15 mm) echogenicity

30. All adnexal masses are ovarian in origin—True or False.

A. True

B. False

C. Partly true

D. Partly false

31. Surgical evaluation is warranted in pelvic masses with:
    A. Abnormal vascularity > 50 mm in size and rising Ca 125
    B. Normal vascularity < 50 mm
    C. Normal vascularity < 30 mm
    D. None of the above

32. In asymptomatic postmenopausal women if the endometrial thickness is 3 mm then next step would be :
    A. TVS every 6 months
    B. Routine ultrasound annually
    C. Endometrial aspiration
    D. Hysteroscopy

33. Factors affecting endometrial thickness on sonography in menopause are:
    A. Time since menopause
    B. Hormone therapy
    C. Tamoxifene therapy for ca breast
    D. Any focal lesion
    E. All of the above

Answer Key

1. A	7. D	13. D	19. C	25. C	31. A
2. A	8. E	14. C	20. F	26. D	32. B
3. D	9. B	15. C	21. A	27. A	33. E
4. A	10. D	16. A	22. A	28. B	
5. B	11. D	17. B	23. B	29. B	
6. D	12. A	18. D	24. A	30. B	

Explanations

5. **B** POI is a spectrum disorder and is a continuum of impaired ovarian function. We define occult POI as impaired ovarian responsiveness to exogenous or endogenous gonadotropin stimulation despite the presence of regular and predictable ovulatory menstrual cycles. Overt POI refers to the presence of irregular menses, elevated serum gonadotropins, and reduced fertility. Gonadotropins will be fluctuating.

6. **D** FSH is not necessary, AMH also not necessary if fertility is not an issue. Thyroid disorders are more common at this age hence TSH is recommended.

7. **D** Bone turnover markers are used only for monitoring response to treatment and do not form the basic investigation at menopause.

13. **D** Advantages of 2d USG are easily available, affordable, in addition to tumor characteristic, can visualize other ovary, enlarged para-aortic nodes, ascitis, other intra-abdominal viscera can be visualized. Doppler differentiates benign from malignancy.

14. **C** For diagnosis of retroperitoneal and intraperitoneal metastasis CT is an excellent modality. Ct is useful in evaluating ovarian masses. MRI-delineates parametrial and myometrial infiltration. Surgery is the 1st line. Not necessary to do fine needle aspiration.

15. **C** Based upon this rationale and the available evidence: For women with BRCA mutations who have completed childbearing, we recommend rrBSO rather than ovarian or fallopian tubal cancer screening or chemoprevention. BSO is advised for women with BRCA mutations regardless of age at diagnosis. The risk for BRCA1 increases linearly with age and remains high even in women who are 50 years or older and have not yet developed ovarian cancer. With regard to BRCA2, the risk does not really climb until women are in their mid–50s. Women with Lynch syndrome should also undergo hysterectomy due to their markedly increased risk of endometrial cancer.

    Clinical practice guidelines Indian menopause society 2015:

    General Recommendations:

    Preventive health screening for healthy post-menopausal women

    A. Annually: BMI, breast examination and pelvic screening for STDs when appropriate. Lipid profile, immunisation counselling for nutrition, physical activities injury prevention, marital and parenteral problems.

    B. Complete medical history and physical examination every 5 years, start at 40 years.

    C. Height-decrease is associated with early osteoporosis. Bone mass should be measured in postmenopausal women who present with fractures, one or more risk factors or >65 years.

    D. TSH–in 40s. Every 2 years from 60 years. Hypothyroidism increases with age and more common in women.

    E. Annual screening mammography from the age of 40.

    F. Colonoscopy at 50 and 55 years. If it is negative and no H/o inherited cancers. no need to repeat.

References

1. Executive summary of the third report of the National Cholesterol Education Program (NCEP) Expert Panel on Detection, Evaluation, and Treatment of High Blood Cholesterol In Adults (Adult Treatment Panel III). JAMA 285:2486–97, 2001.

2. Clinical practice guidelines Indian menopause society 2015 Jaypee.

3. Breast cancer risk assessment and screening in average-risk women. Practice Bulletin No. 179. American College of Obstetricians and Gynecologists. Obstet Gynecol 2017; 130:e1–16.

24. Mehraj Sheikh, Sukhpal Sawhney, Ashok Khurana and Majda Al-Yatama (2009) Alteration of sonographic texture of the endometrium in postmenopausal bleeding a guide to further management, Acta Obstetricia et Gynecologica Scandinavica, 79:11, 1006–10, DOI: 10.1080/00016340009169250

25. Gupta JK, Chien PF, Voit D, Clark TJ, Khan KS. Ultrasonographic endometrial thickness for diagnosing endometrial pathology in women with postmenopausal bleeding: a metaanalysis. Acta Obstet Gynecol Scand 2002; 81: 799–816.

Calcium

◼ *Kanchan Sorte*

1. Hypercalcemia has been reported when daily dose of vitamin D exceeds:
   A. 8000 IU/day
   B. 10000 IU/day
   C. 5000 IU/day
   D. 2000 IU/day

2. Calcium carbonate provides the highest percentage of calcium (40%):
   A. True
   B. False

3. Which calcium salt has least bio-availability?
   A. Calcium citrate
   B. Calcium carbonate
   C. Calcium citrate maleate
   D. Oyster shell calcium

4. What is the recommended allowance of calcium intake in postmenopausal women?
   A. < 500 mg
   B. 500–1000 mg
   C. 1000–1500 mg
   D. > 1500 mg

5. Calcium is not essential in:
   A. Nerve transmission
   B. Muscle contraction
   C. Blood clotting
   D. Cognitive function

6. With low calcium levels which hormone is secreted?
   A. Oestrogen
   B. Progesterone
   C. Parathyroid hormones
   D. Prolactin

7. Calcium supplementation is most useful to prevent:
   A. Alzheimer's
   B. Osteoporosis
   C. CVD
   D. Stroke

8. Peak bone mass is achieved at:
   A. 10–15 years
   B. 25–35 years
   C. 35–45 years
   D. 45–55 years

9. Which vitamin is required for absorption of calcium?
   A. Vitamin A
   B. Vitamin E
   C. Vitamin D
   D. Vitamin C

10. Calcium should not be taken with:
    A. Iron
    B. Analgesics
    C. Vitamin D
    D. Multivitamins

11. Which of the following is not a key player for bone health?
    A. Iron
    B. Vitamin D
    C. Calcium
    D. Vitamin K

12. Richest dietary sources of calcium is:
    A. Green leafy vegetables
    B. Dairy products
    C. Meat
    D. Fish

13. Which factors are important for absorption of calcium?
    A. Solubility of product
    B. Dose/number of doses
    C. Co-ingested food and medication
    D. All of the above

14. Benefits of calcium supplementation include:
    A. Building of bone strength
    B. Reduction in blood pressure
    C. Prevent tooth loss
    D. All of the above

15. Which calcium preparation has toxic levels of lead?
    A. Calcium carbonate
    B. Oyster shell calcium
    C. Calcium citrate
    D. Calcium gluconate

16. Which of the following factors will not cause bone depletion?
    A. Physical activity
    B. Alcohol

C. Tobacco
D. Caffine

17. High doses of calcium supplementation can lead to:
    A. Constipation
    B. Renal stones
    C. Cardiovascular disease
    D. All of the above

18. In which of the following condition calcium levels are depleted:
    A. Menopause
    B. Hyperparathyroidism
    C. Malnutrition/malabsorption
    D. All of the above

19. Calcium taken in divided doses is more beneficial:
    A. True
    B. False

20. Chewable calcium is better tolerated and absorbed:
    A. True
    B. False

21. Calcium supplementation can replace other osteoporosis treatment:
    A. True
    B. False

22. Risk of cardiovascular disease and calculi is not associated with recommended dose calcium.
    A. True
    B. False

Answer Key

1. B	5. D	9. C	13. D	17. D	21. B
2. A	6. C	10. A	14. D	18. D	22. A
3. B	7. B	11. A	15. B	19. A	
4. C	8. B	12. B	16. A	20. A	

Vitamin D

◻ *Ashwini Bhalerao-Gandhi*

1. Upper acceptable limit for daily treatment with vitamin D should not exceed:
   A. 1000 IU/day
   B. 2000 IU/day
   C. 3000 IU/day
   D. 4000 IU/day

2. Groups at higher risk of having low vitamin D are all except:
   A. Infants and young children < 4 years
   B. Pregnant and breastfeeding women
   C. Older people aged 65 years and above
   D. People with low exposure to sun
   E. People who have lighter skin

3. Vitamin D synthesized in the skin is:
   A. Cholecalciferol (vitamin D$_3$)
   B. Ergocalciferol (vitamin D$_2$)
   C. Calcitriol
   D. 7-dehydrocholesterol

4. Sun exposure required for sufficient vitamin D synthesis in skin is:
   A. Sun exposure between 10 am–3 pm for 5–30 minutes at least twice a week providing UVB radiation of wavelength 290–320 nm
   B. Sun exposure between 6 am–8 am for 60 minutes everyday providing UVB radiation of wavelength 340–400 nm
   C. Sun exposure between 7 am–10 am for 60–120 minutes three to four times a week providing UVA radiation of wavelength 270–300 nm
   D. Sun exposure between 12 pm–1 pm everyday for 45 minutes providing UVA radiation of wavelength 360–420 nm

5. Highest concentration of vitamin D is in:
   A. Egg yolk
   B. Tuna fish
   C. Salmon
   D. Peanuts and almonds
   E. Full cream milk

6. Vitamin D insufficiency is defined as 25(OH) D levels:
   A. Between 30 and 40 nmol/ml
   B. Between 20 and 30 ng/ml
   C. Between 10 and 20 nmol/ml
   D. Between 5 and 10 ng/ml

7. Vitamin D deficiency is associated with all except:
   A. Cardiovascular disease
   B. Type 1 diabetes mellitus
   C. Cancer
   D. Psoriasis
   E. Renal stones

8. Skeletal effects of vitamin D deficiency are:
   A. Osteomalacia
   B. Osteopenia
   C. Osteoporosis
   D. All of the above

9. Vitamin D deficiency will result in:
   A. Secondary hyperparathyroidism
   B. Primary hyperparathyroidism
   C. Secondary hypoparathyroidism
   D. Primary hypoparathyroidism

10. Active form of vitamin D is:
    A. Calcitriol
    B. Cholecalciferol
    C. Ergocalciferol
    D. 7 dehydrocholesterol

11. Major circulating and storage form of vitamin D is:
    A. 1 Hydroxy vitamin D
    B. 25 hydroxy vitamin D
    C. 1, 25 dihydroxy vitamin D
    D. Calcitriol

12. Vitamin D is converted to its biologically active form in:
    A. Liver
    B. Lung
    C. Kidney
    D. Duodenum

13. Which statement is false:
    A. Vitamin D_2 is known as ergocalciferol and is of plant source
    B. Vitamin D_3 is known as cholecalciferol and is of animal source
    C. Vitamin D_3 has more biological activity than vitamin D_2
    D. Vitamin D_2 and vitamin D_3 are activated equally by vitamin D hydroxylases

14. Gynaecological disorder strongly associated with vitamin D deficiency is:
    A. PCOS
    B. Premenstrual syndrome
    C. Uterine fibroids
    D. Endometriosis

15. Indications for BMD testing in post-menopausal women:
    A. All women aged 65 years and above regardless of clinical risk factors
    B. Postmenopausal women > 50 years and thin
    C. Postmenopausal women > 50 years and smokers
    D. Postmenopausal women > 50 years and with Rheumatoid arthritis
    E. All of the above

16. Vitamin D is available as:
    A. Oily solution in capsule
    B. Sachets
    C. Micellised form
    D. All of the above

17. 70 years old woman has fracture neck femur. Her vitamin D is 7. How will you manage?
    A. Let orthopedic decide. Not my problem
    B. Vitamin D sachets, 60.000 daily for 1 month then weekly
    C. Vitamin D injection 6 lakhs stat, then sachets/capsules weekly
    D. Vitamin D injection 6 lakhs stat, then Micellised form weekly
    E. Check calcium/PTH/kidney function/dexa before planning therapy.

18. Match the following:

Column A		Column B	
A.	Rickets	i.	CT scan
B.	Osteomalacia	ii.	Excess intake of calcium
C.	Osteoporosis	iii.	Menopause
D.	Kidney stones	iv.	Multiparity
E.	Parathyroid tumor	v.	Children

19. Causes of hypervitaminosis D include all except:
    A. Excess exposure to sunlight
    B. Hodgkin's lymphoma
    C. MEN-L
    D. Sarcoidosis

20. Drugs which affect vitamin D metabolism are:
   A. Antiepileptics
   B. Cholestyramine
   C. Prednisolone
   D. All of the above

21. Why is vitamin D so low in Indian population:
   A. Desire to avoid sun for fair skin
   B. Poverty and poor nutritional status
   C. Women are fully covered in garments
   D. All of the above

Answer Key

1. D	9. A	17. E
2. E	10. A	18. A v
3. A	11. B	B iv
4. A	12. C	C iii
5. C	13. C	D ii
6. B	14. A	E i
7. E	15. E	19. A
8. D	16. D	20. D
		21. D

Micronutrients other than Calcium and Vitamin D

◼ *Bhumika*

1. Vitamin E as a menopausal health supplement:
   A. High dose helps with hot flushes
   B. Beneficial effects on skin and hair
   C. Helps in muscle function
   D. Dietary sources available

2. Pick the correct statement about concurrent supplementation of calcium, and other micronutrients:
   A. There is no known effect
   B. The phytases hamper absorption of only calcium
   C. No effect on copper retention
   D. Formation of insoluble Zn-Ca-phytase complexes, render Zn unavailable for absorption

3. Percentage of magnesium found in bones is:
   A. 30%
   B. 70%
   C. 10%
   D. 50%

4. Omega 3 in fish oil have following benefits:
   A. Potent anti-inflammatory
   B. Skin and hair benefits
   C. Cardiovascular benefits

   D. Preserves brain function including cognitive delay, dementia and Alzheimer's
   E. All the above

5. Recommended dose of fish oil:
   A. 1000–2000 mg of EPA and DHA daily
   B. 2000–3000 mg of EPA and DHA daily
   C. 3000–4000 mg of EPA and DHA daily
   D. 5000–6000 mg of EPA and DHA daily

6. Compound combined with vitamin C to reduce hot flushes is
   A. Biotin
   B. Hepsin
   C. Inositol
   D. Hesperidin

7. Menopausal herbal supplement includes in all except:
   A. Black cohosh
   B. Red clover
   C. Saint John's wort
   D. Boswellia

8. Which of the following are known to reduce oxidative stress of menopause?
   A. Vitamin C
   B. Vitamin E

C. Physical activity

D. All of the above

9. To overcome insomnia in menopause all can be done, except:

   A. No caffeine at bed time

   B. Magnesium intake

   C. Exercise during day

   D. Vitamins B_6 and B_{12} intake, as it produces serotonin

10. Menopausal supplement for osteoporosis is:

   A. Calcium

   B. Black cohosh

   C. Cnidium monnieri

   D. All of the above

11. Vitamin E prevents coronary arterial disease by:

   A. Potent antioxidant and platelet aggregation inhibition

   B. Reducing calcium absorption and retention

   C. Maintaining metabolism of homocystiene

   D. None of the above

12. Magnesium deficiency impairs:

   A. Parathyroid hormone secretion

   B. Growth hormone

   C. Glucocorticoids

   D. Thyroid hormone

13. Magnesium intake sufficient to maintain magnesium reserve is:

   A. 300 mg

   B. 200 mg

   C. 600 mg

   D. 800 mg

Answer Key

1. C	4. E	7. D	10. D	13. A
2. D	5. A	8. B	11. A	
3. D	6. D	9. D	12. A	

Reference

Purandare CN, Suvarna Khadilkar. chapter 10 Menopause: Current Concepts: 2004, Jaypee under auspices of FOGSI.

Diet in Menopause

◙ *Shefali Kamal Kumar*

1. What is one of the major dietary requirements of menopause?
   A. Increased caloric consumption
   B. Decreased empty caloric consumption
   C. Decreased proteins

2. The protein requirements increase in menopause due to which of the following reasons?
   A. To help reduce the weight gained
   B. To help reduce the effects of muscle loss initiated by the decline in estrogen
   C. Both A and B

3. What is the richest vegan source of calcium?
   A. Milk
   B. Ragi
   C. Cheese

4. Which is the cheapest and richest source of vitamin D?
   A. Sunlight
   B. Eggs
   C. Wheat

5. Why is iron an essential nutrient for the Indian menopausal woman?
   A. Because it generally declines during menopause
   B. Because most Indian women suffer from anemia

C. Because most Indian women consume high amounts of calcium

6. Which of the following vitamin(s) are/is essential to alleviate the dry skin problem of menopause?
   A. Vitamin K
   B. Vitamin B_6
   C. Vitamin E

7. What is the ideal rate of weight loss in menopause?
   A. 5 kilos per month
   B. Half a kilo per w
   C. 2 kilos per week

8. Besides proteins, which is one of the most essential nutrients in the fight against weight gain?
   A. Fats
   B. Vitamin K
   C. Fiber

9. Phytoestrogens share the structural similarity to which estrogen form?
   A. Estrone
   B. Estriol
   C. Estradiol

10. What are the commonly found sources of phytoestrogens in the Indian diet?
    A. Soy and its products
    B. Fenugreek and Oats
    C. Both A and B

11. Carbohydrate rich foods can help improve one's mood. Is this statement True or False?
    A. True
    B. False

12. Which is the food that has shown to decrease hot flashes in menopausal women?
    A. Iced beverages
    B. Tea and coffee
    C. Soy and its products

13. What can be used as an effective sleep aid for menopausal women?
    A. Warm milk with bournvita
    B. Warm milk with nutmeg and cinnamon
    C. Warm milk with haldi and sugar

14. Which of the following is generally used as a CAM in menopause?
    A. Black pepper
    B. Black salt
    C. Black cohosh

15. Kava is known to cause which of the following problems?
    A. Hepatic problems
    B. Seizures
    C. Affects clotting times

16. Which of the following is responsible for the psychological disturbances during menopause?
    A. Altered appearance
    B. Depression, stress, anxiety
    C. All of the above

17. State whether the following is true or false: It is possible to follow an ideal diet.
    A. True
    B. False

18. State whether the following is true or false: Meats should be recommended liberally during menopause as they are rich in proteins and calcium.
    A. True
    B. False

19. State whether the following is true or false: Vitamin D may help combat depression.
    A. True
    B. False

20. State whether the following is true or false: Spot reduction is possible via diet.
    A. True
    B. False

21. After the age of 30 years the calorie required decreases every decade by about:
    A. 10%
    B. 20%
    C. 30%
    D. 35%

22. Dietary prescription for postmenopausal women should contain all except:
    A. Complex carbohydrates inclu-ding fibres
    B. Barley
    C. Fermented foods
    D. Refined carbohydrates

23. Postmenopausal depressive symptoms are not alleviated by balanced diet and triptophan rich food.
    A. True
    B. False

Answer Key

1. B	5. B	9. C	13. B	17. B	21. A
2. C	6. C	10. C	14. C	18. B	22. D
3. B	7. B	11. A	15. A	19. A	23. B
4. A	8. C	12. C	16. C	20. B	

Explanations

1. **B** Decreased empty caloric consumption (due to a reduction in the resting metabolic rate as a result of aging and decreased activity levels due to various physiological and psychological reasons).

2. **C** Both A and B (proteins help in reducing the weight of the menopausal lady while ensuring adequate muscle build-up).

3. **B**. Ragi (the other two options are vegetarian options).

4. **A** Sunlight (sunlight is available for free everywhere with a minimum of forty minute exposure daily).

5. **B** Because most Indian women suffer from anemia (even though menopause sees no significant decline in the levels of iron in women internationally, Indian women have an extremely high prevalence of anemia, making iron and essential nutrient).

6. **C** Vitamin E (vitamin E helps in reducing dry skin when taken orally and topically).

7. **B** Half a kilo per week (a rate higher than this is not only difficult to sustain in the long run, but also is difficult to maintain once the weight loss target has been achieved).

8 **C** Fiber (fiber is essential as it promotes weight loss, a reduction in the lipid levels and blood glucose levels and relieves constipation).

10. **C** Both A and B (other sources include apples, anise seeds, mint, flax seeds, etc.).

11. **A** True (carbohydrate rich foods can improve the levels of serotonin according to some studies).

12. **C** Soy and its products (soy has phytoestrogenic properties that help reduce hot flashes).

17. **B** False (it is only possible to follow an ideal diet under ideal conditions which are generally not possible in daily life).

18. **B** False (meats are known to cause problems like hypercholesterolemia, hypertriglyceridemia, hyperuricemia, etc. and hence need to be recommended prudent.

20. **B** False (spot reduction is only possible via surgery because when weight loss occurs, it happens all over the body).

Yoga/Exercise in Menopause

◼ *Madhuri Mehendale*

1. The exercise program for postmeno-pausal women should include:
   A. The endurance exercise (aerobic)
   B. Strength exercise
   C. Balance exercise
   D. All of the above

2. The exercise program for postmeno-pausal women should aim for:
   A. At least two hours and 30 minutes of moderate aerobic activity each week
   B. As per ones capacity
   C. Depends on ones heart rate
   D. One hour daily

3. All are true except:
   A. Even if the BMD is not improved as measured by the dexascan, resistance training with adequate intensity will dramatically lower the lifetime fracture risk
   B. If high load and low rep routines of compound exercises are used, these stimulate muscle develop-ment around the hips, spine, and arms, building bone strength
   C. The frequency of load is most relevant in BMD changes, not the maximal load
   D. It can take four to six months or more for the bone to remodel

under the best conditions, and the measurable effects of exercise may only be apparent years later

4. To determine the maximum heart rate for exercise:
   A. One has to subtract the woman's age from 220
   B. Multiply heart rate by 80/100
   C. Multiply heart rate by 50/100
   D. One has to subtract the woman's age from 200

5. The current recommendations for non pharmacological management of menopausal symptoms are:
   A. Change in lifestyle and diet
   B. Regular exercise
   C. Yoga, therapeutic massage and other stress-reducing measures
   D. All of the above

6. Yoga improves sleeping pattern by:
   A. Increasing plasma melatonin levels
   B. Increasing physical excretion and exhaustion
   C. Unknown mechanism
   D. Increasing mental balance

7. Pranayama helps in menopausal symptoms by strengthens the lungs:
   A. Slows down mental chatter and infuses positive thinking

B. Improves their function and enhances the lung power

C. It improves the defense mechanism of the body

D. All of the above

8. All is true about yoga in menopausal period except:
   A. Provides distraction from daily life
   B. Reduce anxiety, depression
   C. Improves hot flushes and night sweats
   D. Improves mental balance, attention and remote memory

9. Weight-bearing exercises include all except:
   A. Cycling
   B. Walking
   C. Jogging
   D. Swimming

10. Aerobic exercises includes all except:
   A. Walking
   B. Swimming
   C. Yoga
   D. Cycling

Answer Key

1. D	3. C	5. D	7. D	9. D
2. A	4. A	6. A	8. C	10. C

References

1. J Midlife Health. 2011 Jul-Dec; 2(2): 51–56. Exercise beyond menopause: Dos and Don'ts. Nalini Mishra, VN Mishra,[1] and Devanshi[2]
2. J Midlife Health. 2010 Jul-Dec; 1(2): 56–58. Yoga and menopausal transition Nirmala Vaze and Sulabha Joshi.

Chapter

13

Sexuality and Menopause

◉ *Madhuri Mehendale*

1. Menopause is associated with physiological and psychological changes that influence sexuality: the primary biological change is:
   A. A decrease in circulating estrogen levels
   B. Decrease in testosterone levels to less than 50%
   C. Decrease in progesterone
   D. Nonhormonal

2. Continual estrogen loss during menopause is associated with:
   A. Changes in the vascular, muscular, and urogenital systems
   B. Alterations in mood, sleep, and cognitive functioning
   C. Decreased sexual function
   D. All of the above

3. Nonhormonal factors that affect sexuality are:
   A. Health status and current medication use
   B. Changes in or dissatisfaction with partner
   C. Socioeconomic status
   D. All of the above

4. All of the below can be used for FSD in menopause except:
   A. Systemic estrogen

B. Tibolone
C. SERMS
D. Systemic testosterone

5. Anatomical changes seen during menopause are:
   A. Vaginal vault becomes pale in appearance and less elastic with loss of rugation
   B. Tissue friability followed by progressive shortening and narrowing
   C. The clitoris gets fibrosed and the vulvar and labial tissues lose fullness
   D. All of the above

6. The factors affecting sexual function during menopause are:
   A. Prior level of sexual function
   B. Change in partner status and feelings for partner
   C. Estradiol level
   D. All of the above

7. Female sexual disorders is defined as:
   A. Four diagnostic groups: desire, arousal, orgasm and pain problems
   B. Two diagnostic groups: orgasm and arousal
   C. Orgasmic problems
   D. Decreased sexual desire

8. Sildenafil works best in women with:
   A. Arousal disorders
   B. Decreased desire
   C. Pain
   D. Orgasm

9. Testosterone therapy in the low-dose regimens is efficacious for the treatment of:
   A. Women's sexual interest and desire disorder in postmenopausal women who are adequately estrogenized

   B. Pain
   C. Arousal disorder
   D. Should not be used

10. Women with decreased libido inspite of adequate estrogen/progesterone therapy can be treated with:
   A. Testosterone
   B. Sildenafil
   C. Tibolone
   D. Aromatase inhibitors

Answer Key

1. A	3. D	5. D	7. A	9. A
2. D	4. D	6. D	8. A	10. C

References

3. **D** Reference for 1 to 3,Graziottin A, Leiblum SR. Biological and psychosocial pathophysiology of female sexual dysfunction during the menopausal transition. J Sex Med 2005; 2(suppl 3):133–45.

4,5. **D** Continuing medical education: The use of estrogen therapy in women's sexual functioning (CME) Rossella E. Nappi MD, PhD; Franco Polatti MD.

6. **D** Dennerstein L, Lehert P, Burger H. The relative effects of hormones and relationship factors on sexual function of women through the natural menopausal transition. Fertil Steril 2005; 84:174–80.

7,8. **A** Sexual dysfunction in the peri- and post-menopause. Status of incidence, pharmacological treatment and possible risks. A secondary publication.Gregersen N1, Jensen PT, Giraldi AE.

9. **A** Int J Impot Res. 2005 Sep-Oct; 17(5):399–408.Testosterone therapy in women: a review.Bolour S1, Braunstein G.

10. **C** Menopause. 2002 May-Jun; 9(3):162–70.The effects of tibolone on mood and libido. Davis SR1.

Fertility Issues at Menopause

◉ *Punit Bhojani*

INFERTILITY ISSUES AT PERIMENOPAUSE

1. AMH levels which indicate very low fertility is _____ ng/ml
   A. > 6.5
   B. 2–4
   C. 0.3–2
   D. < 0.3

2. Best marker for ovarian reserve is:
   A. FSH
   B. USG
   C. AMH
   D. FSH/LH ratio

3. In woman with diminished ovarian reserve this drug can be used:
   A. Prednisolone
   B. Heparin
   C. DHEA
   D. Aspirin

4. DHEA benefits are:
   A. Increased IVF pregnancy rates
   B. Increased chance of spontaneous conceptions
   C. Increased quality and quantity of eggs and embryos
   D. All of the above

5. A 45-year-old woman who had two normal pregnancies 15 and 18 years ago presents with the complaint of amenorrhea for 7 months. She expresses the desire to become pregnant again. After exclusion of pregnancy, which of the following is the next best test indicated in the evaluation of this patient's amenorrhea?
   A. LH and FSH levels
   B. Endometrial biopsy
   C. Karyotyping
   D. HSG

6. In an amenorrheic patient who has had pituitary ablation for a craniopharyngioma, which of the following regimens is most likely to result in an ovulatory cycle?
   A. Clomiphene citrate
   B. Letrozole
   C. Continuous infusion of GnRH
   D. Human menopausal or recombinant gonadotropin, followed by hCG

7. Best indicator for ovarian reserve among these is:
   A. LH
   B. LH/FSH ratio
   C. FSH
   D. Estradiol

8. AMH is measured on which day of the cycle:
   A. Day 2
   B. Day 14
   C. Day 21
   D. Any day of the cycle

9. An infertile woman has bilateral tubal block at cornua diagnosed on hysterosalpingography. Next treatment of choice is:
   A. IVF
   B. Laparoscopy and hysteroscopy
   C. Tuboplasty
   D. Hydrotubation

10. True about Swyer syndrome:
    A. 46XX
    B. Infertility treated with IVF and surrogacy
    C. Infertility treated with IVF and donor oocyte
    D. Gonadectomy not indicated

11. AMH/MIS is secreted by:
    A. Leydig cells
    B. Sertoli cells
    C. Theca cells
    D. All of the above

12. Test used to detect genetic abnormality in embryo, before transferring it to the uterus in IVF is:
    A. Embryo cell biopsy
    B. CVS
    C. ICSI
    D. All of the above

13. Oldest woman in history to give birth was at the age of:
    A. 50 years
    B. 60 years
    C. 70 years
    D. 80 years

14. A surrogate mother should not be over _____ years of age:
    A. 35
    B. 45
    C. 50
    D. 55

15. The problem with elderly women undergoing ART are:
    A. Oocytes are of poorer quality
    B. The zona pellucida is thickened
    C. Higher incidence of chromosomal abnormalities
    D. All of the above

16. Options available for infertility issues at perimenopause are:
    A. Egg donation
    B. Embryo donation
    C. Adoption
    D. All of the above

17. As the fecundity declines with age monthly chances of conceiving at 40 years declines to:
    A. 2%
    B. 30%
    C. 8%
    D. 18%

18. Controlled ovarian hyperstimulation is the treatment of choice for women with primary and secondary premature ovarian failure.
    A. True
    B. False

Answer Key

1. D	5. A	9. B	13. C	17. C
2. C	6. D	10. C	14. B	18. B
3. C	7. C	11. B	15. D	
4. D	8. D	12. A	16. D	

Explanantions

1. **D** AMH levels (ng/mL) Interpretation
   4.0–6.8 Optimal fertility
   2.2–4.0 Satisfactory fertility
   0.3–2.2 Low fertility
   < 0.3 Very low fertility
   > 6.8 High levels (PCOS and granulosa cell tumor)

2. **C** AMH or anti-Müllerian hormone is a substance that is produced by granulosa cells in ovarian follicles. It is first made in primary follicles that advance from the primordial follicle stage. At these stages, follicles are microscopic and cannot be seen by ultrasound. AMH production is highest in pre-antral and small antral stages (< 4 mm diameter) of follicle development.
   Since AMH is produced only in small ovarian follicles, blood levels of AMH have been used to measure the size of the pool of growing follicles.
   Research shows that the size of the pool of growing follicles is greatly influenced by the size of the pool of remaining primordial follicles (microscopic follicles in 'deep sleep').
   Hence, AMH blood levels are thought to reflect the size of the remaining egg supply or 'ovarian reserve'.

3. **C** Dehydroepiandrosterone (DHEA) 25 mg three times a day for 3 months has been reported to improve pregnancy chances in patients with Diminished Ovarian Reserve which occurs either as a consequence of premature ovarian aging (POA) or female aging.
   DHEA is a naturally existing hormone that the female body converts into androgens, mainly testosterone. Even though androgens are male hormones, they are present in both sexes and are essential in the female body for the production and development of healthy eggs.

4. **D** DHEA's beneficial effects on female fertility include:
   1. Increased IVF pregnancy rates
   2. Increased chance of spontaneous conceptions
   3. Shortened time to pregnancy
   4. Increased quality and quantity of eggs and embryos
   5. Decreased risk of miscarriage and chromosomal abnormalities in embryos
   6. Improved cumulative pregnancy rates in patients under fertility treatment.

5. **A** (LH and FSH levels): This patient has secondary amenorrhea, which rules out abnormalities associated with primary amenorrhea such as congenital Müllerian abnormalities and chromosomal abnormalities. The most common cause for secondary amenorrhea in a woman of reproductive age is pregnancy, which should be evaluated first. Other possibilities include chronic endometritis or scarring of the endometrium (Asherman's syndrome), hypothyroidism, and ovarian failure. The latter is the most likely diagnosis in a woman at this age. In addition, extreme weight loss, emotional stress and adrenal cortisol insufficiency can bring about secondary amenorrhea. A HSG is part of an infertility workup that may demonstrate Asherman syndrome, but it is not indicated until premature ovarian failure has been excluded. Persistently elevated gonadotropin levels (especially when accompanied by low serum estradiol levels) are diagnostic of ovarian failure.

6. **D** (Human menopausal or recombinant gonadotropin, followed by hCG): This patient will not be able to produce endogenous gonadotropin, since her pituitary has been ablated. The patient will, therefore, need to be given exogenous gonadotropin in the form of human menopausal gonadotropin (hMG), which contains an extract of urine from postmenopausal women with FSH and LH in various ratio for follicular growth. Recombinant FSH is now also available. Timed administration of hCG, which takes the place of an endogenous LH surge, will be needed to complete oocyte maturation and induce ovulation.
   Clomiphene citrate and letrozole block the normal negative feedback of the endogenous estrogens and stimulates release of endogenous GnRH and FSH, but this will not be helpful as the patient's pituitary has been ablated. Similarly, endogenous or exogenous GnRH cannot stimulate the release of FSH or LH in this woman because the pituitary gland is nonfunctional.

8. **D** AMH test can be done on any day of a woman's cycle unlike FSH level test, which has to be done on day 2 or 3 of the menstrual cycle.

9. **B** (Laparoscopy and hysteroscopy)
   In hysterosalpingography (HSG), cavity of the uterus and fallopian tube patency can be checked.
   - As it does not require anesthesia, it is the first-line investigation for checking tubal patency.
   - *Disadvantage:* While pushing the dye, there can be cornual spasm and the fallopian tubes can appear to be blocked even if the tubes are normal/healthy. So HSG cannot differentiate between cornual blocks (pathological) and cornual spasm.
   - Laparoscopy (with chromopertubation with methylene blue dye): Best investigation for tubal patency, as tubal patency be confirmed under vision, and besides, any pathology can simultaneously be corrected with operative laparoscopy.
   - This patient has bilateral cornual blocks on HSG, and hence, a laparoscopy should be done to confirm the findings.
   - If on laparoscopy there is a presence of cornual block, cornual catheterization (using operative hysteroscopy) should be done simultaneously to remove the blocks.
   - IVF is the option in inoperable cases/severely damaged tubes or if surgery fails to remove the blocks.

10. **C** (Infertility treated with IVF and donor oocyte)
    Swyer syndrome is XY pure gonadal dysgenesis.
    The syndrome was named by Gerald Swyer, an endocrinologist, based in London.
    Swyer syndrome occurs in approximately 1 in 80,000 people.
    Patient with Swyer syndrome have typical female external genitalia and are typically raised as girls and have a female gender identity but the karyotype is 46XY.
    The uterus and fallopian tubes are formed, but the gonads are not functional; affected individuals have undeveloped clumps of tissue called streak gonads.
    Without testes, testosterone and AMH both are not produced. Without testosterone, the wolffian ducts fail to develop, so no internal male organs are formed. Also, the lack of testosterone means that no dihydrotestosterone is formed and so the external genitalia fail to virilize, resulting in normal female genitalia. Since AMH is absent the Müllerian ducts develop into normal internal female organs (uterus, fallopian tubes, cervix, vagina).
    Because they lack ovaries, girls with Swyer syndrome do not produce sex hormones and will not undergo puberty (unless treated with hormone replacement therapy).
    As they do not have functional ovaries, affected individuals usually require hormone replacement therapy during adolescence to induce menstruation and development of female secondary sex characteristics such as breast enlargement and uterine growth. Hormone replacement therapy also helps reduce the risk of osteopenia and osteoporosis.
    Women with this disorder cannot have their own biological child as they do not produce ova but they can become pregnant with IVF and Donor Oocyte. As uterus is present surrogacy is not required.
    The residual gonadal tissue often becomes cancerous, so it is usually removed surgically early in life.
    Streak gonads are usually removed within a year or so of diagnosis since the cancer (gonadoblstoma) can begin during infancy.

11. **B** (Sertoli cells)
    Mullerian inhibiting substance (MIS)/Anti-Müllerian hormone (AMH) is the gonadal hormone that causes regression of the Müllerian ducts, during male embryogenesis.
    MIS is a member of the large transforming growth factor-β (TGF-β) multigene family of glycoproteins that are involved in the regulation of growth and differentiation.
    AMH in males is secreted by Sertoli cells.
    Testosterone is secreted from Leydig cells.
    In females, AMH is produced by granulosa cells in ovarian follicles and is a marker for ovarian reserve.

12. **A** (Embryo cell biopsy)

Preimplantation genetic diagnosis (PGD) is a reproductive technology used with an IVF cycle. As the name suggests, it can be used for preimplantation diagnosis of genetic disease in embryos.

PGD, involves removing a cell from an IVF embryo to test it for a specific genetic condition (e.g. cystic fibrosis) before transferring the embryo to the uterus.

When used to screen for a specific genetic disease, its main advantage is that it avoids MTP, as the method makes it highly likely that the baby will be free of the disease.

PGD facilitates DNA study of the eggs or embryos to find out those that carry mutations for genetic diseases. It is useful in cases having a history of chromosomal or genetic disorders in the family.

13. **C** Daljinder Kaur (from India) who's believed to be at least 70 years old, gave birth to a son named Arman. The baby was the first for Kaur and her 79-year-old husband, Mohinder Singh Gill, after nearly five decades of marriage.

14. **B** A surrogate mother should not be over 45 years of age. Before accepting a woman as a possible surrogate for a particular couple's child, the ART clinic must ensure (and put on record) that the woman satisfies all the testable criteria to go through a successful full-term pregnancy.

Contraception

◙ *Deepali Prakash Kale*

1. The accurate marker for fertility cessation at menopause transition is:
   A. High FSH > 40 IU
   B. Serum estradiol < 20 pg/ml
   C. No biological marker exist
   D. Low AMH

2. Mrs XY 52-year-old female using non-hormonal contraception. She had no periods since 1 year. How long she should continue contraceptive use:
   A. Immediately stop contraception
   B. Continue for 6 months
   C. Continue for 2 years
   D. Continue for 1 year

3. In women using COC (combined oral contraceptive) it is well known fact that COC affects FSH levels. The recommended period for which COC needs to be stopped prior to testing the FSH level is:
   A. 1 week
   B. 2 weeks
   C. 3 weeks
   D. 4 weeks

4. Regarding MHT and contraception all are true except:
   A. MHT inhibits ovulation in only 40% of users
   B. Progesterone only pills are suitable for the MHT users
   C. IUCD are suitable
   D. In non-hysterectomised women combined hormonal contraceptive pills (E+P) the progesterone component provides endometrial protection

5. Risk of venous thromboembolism after starting using the hormonal contraception is maximum in:
   A. 1 month
   B. 6 months
   C. 2 years
   D. 4 months

6. Following is contraindicated in perimenopausal age group:
   A. Progesterone only pill
   B. High dose estrogen combined OC pill
   C. LNG-IUS
   D. None of the above

7. Most suitable option in perimenopausal women suffering from menorrhagia is:
   A. Cu-T
   B. Injectable DMPA
   C. Low dose oral contraceptive pill
   D. LNG-IUS

8. Contraception in perimenopause is indicated because:
   A. Pregnancy is associated with increased maternal complication
   B. Pregnancy is associated with increased fetal malformation and complication
   C. Unintended pregnancies are known up to 1 year after menopause
   D. All of the above

9. Perimenopausal women suffering from osteoporosis are not prescribed:
   A. Low dose OC pills
   B. Injectable depo medroxyprogesterone
   C. IUCD
   D. All of the above

10. Goals for contraception in perimenopausal age are:
   A. Prevent pregnancy
   B. Reduce hormonal fluctuations associated with perimenopause
   C. Provide additional non-contraceptive benefits like cancer prevention, bone protection
   D. All of the above

Answer Key

1. C	3. B	5. D	7. D	9. B
2. A	4. D	6. B	8. D	10. D

Checklist before Menopausal Hormone Therapy (MHT)
(History, Examination, Investigation)

◉ *Suvarna Khadilkar*

1. **When will you prescribe MHT?**
   A. Hot flushes > 5 times a day
   B. Insomnia at least once in a month
   C. Quality of life compromised
   D. All of the above

2. **MHT can be started in all of the following except:**
   A. Atrophic vaginitis
   B. Recurrent UTI with no other cause identified
   C. High-risk for osteoporosis related fractures
   D. Women beyond ten years of menopause or age > 60 years

3. **State true or false: Following advice is given as caution and for follow-up while on MHT:**
   A. Dexa test is mandatory before starting MHT
   B. One year amenorrhoea is a must before starting tibolone
   C. An annual follow-up with mammography is must in all patients
   D. The dose and duration of HT individualized and must start with smallest possible dose
   E. A risk benefit assessment carried out annually or earlier if new symptoms emerge

   F. A full gynecological assessment mandatory prior to starting HT and at regular intervals thereafter
   G. Clinical breast examination should be done monthly
   H. A mammogram [where available] –1–3 yearly if the initial mammogram is normal

4. **Following are considered relative contraindications except:**
   A. Porphyria cutanea tarda
   B. Migraine headaches
   C. Active gallbladder disease (cholangitis, cholecystitis)
   D. History of uterine fibroids

5. **Common side effects of combined MHT all except:**
   A. Headache
   B. Upset stomach, stomach cramps or bloating
   C. Diarrhea
   D. Appetite and weight changes
   E. Changes in sex drive or performance
   F. Breast tenderness
   G. Brown or black patches on the skin
   H. Acne
   I. Swelling of hands, feet, or lower legs due to fluid retention

J. Spotting or bleeding per vaginum

K. Breast tenderness, enlargement, or discharge

6. MHT should be discontinued in all situations except:

A. If migraine appears for the first time or if headache gets worsened

B. Blurring of vision or any symptoms suggesting of vascular occlusion

C. If jaundice appears

D. If there is significant rise in blood pressure

E. If an elective surgery is planned after 3 months

Answer Key

1. C	B True	E True	H True	6. E
2. D	C False	F True	4. A	
3. A False	D True	G False	5. E	

Explanations

1. **C** Clinical practice guideline on menopause, executive summary and recommendations, Indian Menopause Society. *J Mid Life Health* 2013.
2. **D** Global consensus international menopause society April 2013, FOGSI statement on MHT, 2014.
3. **C** False. Decision should be individualized.
3. **D** True. One size does not fit all.
3. **G** False. Self breast examination monthly and clinical examination annually recommended.
4. **A** Answer is Porphyria cutanea tarda as this is an absolute contraindication.
5. **E** Changes in sex drive or performance (this is not a side effect but desirable effect).

Menopausal Hormone Therapy

◙ *Seema Sharma*

1. Addition of progesterone to estrogen replacement benefits:
   A. Endometrium
   B. Breast
   C. Heart
   D. All of the above

2. Transdermal administration of estrogen is preferred in women with:
   A. Hypertension
   B. Hypertriglyceridemia
   C. Increased risk for chololithiasis
   D. All of the above

3. Which of the following is true?
   A. Oral MHT is more effective than transdermal methods for relieving vasomotor symptoms
   B. Transdermal hormone therapy is less likely to be associated with stroke and DVT than oral therapy
   C. As compared to low dose MHT, higher doses of MHT are more effective for relieving hot flashes and just as safe
   D. Once started, women should stay on HRT for at least 10 years to avoid the recurrence of any hot flashes

4. MHT causes improvement in menopausal symptoms. Which of the following precaution needs to be taken while on MHT?
   A. Yearly breast mammogram
   B. Yearly brain scans
   C. Yearly lung scans
   D. Yearly hormone profile

5. Pulsed estrogen therapy is given via:
   A. Transnasal route
   B. Transdermal route
   C. Transvaginal route
   D. Oral route

6. HERS (heart estrogen-progesterone replacement study) ended after 4.1 years due to:
   A. It proved efficiency of estrogen as cardioprotective agent
   B. It showed no change in lipid profile of estrogen user
   C. Coronary events increased by 50% during the first year of trial
   D. All of the above

7. The largest study of WHI of estrogen + progesterone therapy, following holds true:
   A. It was a randomized study
   B. It was done on 16,608 subjects
   C. It was halted prematurely in July 2002
   D. All of the above

8. WHI project halted prematurely due to all of the following reasons except:
   A. Increased rate of coronary events in MHT users
   B. Increased incidence of stroke in MHT users
   C. Administration and financial problems
   D. Two fold rise in the risk of venous thromboembolism

9. Which type of progesterone does not have reversal of beneficial effect of estrogen on cardiovascular system?
   A. Medroxy progesterone
   B. Norethisterone
   C. Desogestral
   D. All of the above

10. MHT should be used in lowest possible dose, but exceptions to low dose therapy are all except:
    A. Premature ovarian failure
    B. Dementia
    C. Severe osteoporosis
    D. Climacteric depression

11. Which of the following will cause least hepatic load?
    A. 17 β estradiol
    B. Conjugated equine estrogen
    C. Ethinyl estradiol
    D. All of the above

12. Choose the correct statement regarding potency of various estrogens:
    A. Relative potency for receptor affinity is 100 for ethinyl estradiol. Estradiol has a potency of 20000, estrone has 10 and estriol has 1–5
    B. Based on effect on HDL cholesterol, relative potencies of estradiol 100 estrone 20, estriol 50, ethinyl estradiol 40000
    C. Relative potency for receptor affinity is 10 for ethinyl estradiol. Estradiol has a potency of 20000 estrone has 100 and estriol has 15
    D. None of the above

13. Which of the available hormonal therapies should be preferred in following situations?

    I. Perimenopausal woman hot flushes and insomnia compromising the quality of life with intact uterus
    A. Tibolone

    II. Loss of libido final menstrual period 12 months back
    B. Continuous unopposed estrogen therapy with or without androgens

    III. Symptomatic surgical menopause
    C. Continuous combined estrogen and progesterone therapy

    IV. Postmenopausal woman with intact uterus
    D. Short-term cyclical estrogen and progesterone therapy

14. Which of the following progesterone is not associated with high breast cancer incidence?
    A. Medroxy progesterone
    B. Dydrogesterone
    C. Micronised progesterone
    D. Both B and C are correct

15. A 52 years old Indian woman complaining of dyspareunia, hot flushes, compromising quality of life the best treatment option is:
    A. Local estrogen cream
    B. Transdermal estrogen patches
    C. Oral estrogen therapy
    D. None of the above

Answer Key

1. A	4. A	7. D	10. B	13. I D	IV C
2. D	5. A	8. C	11. A	II A	14. D
3. B	6. C	9. C	12. B	III B	15. C

Explanataion and References

1. Clinical practice guidelines on menopause 2012, updated 2015, Indian Menopause Society
2. Management handbook. Health Plan for the Adult Woman; International Menopause Society
12. Kuhl BH. Pharmacology of estrogens and progestogens: Influence of different routes of administration, climacteric 2005.

18

Menopausal Hormone Therapy (MHT) in High-Risk Cases

◉ *Suvarna Khadilkar*

1. Absolute contraindications for MHT are:
   A. Thromboembolism
   B. Pregnancy
   C. Ca breast, endometrium
   D. All of the above

2. Secondary prevention of cardiovascular disease:
   A. Should be done with MHT
   B. Should be avoided with MHT
   C. Has shown poor results in HERS
   D. B and C both are true

3. WHIM 2003, have described estrogen's role in neuroprotection as:
   A. It worsens memory and cognition
   B. It improves memory and cognition
   C. It prevents Alzheimers
   D. None of the above

4. If MHT use is extended beyond 5 years:
   A. It increases risk of breast cancer
   B. The risk of carcinoma breast remains unaltered
   C. It reduces the risk of breast cancer
   D. None of the above

5. Prognosis of Ca breast secondary to MHT as compared to primary Ca breast:
   A. Worse
   B. Similar
   C. Better
   D. Cannot say

6. Patient suffering from diabetes mellitus following drug is preferred for MHT:
   A. Estrogen and progestogen
   B. Tibolone
   C. None of the two A and B
   D. No drug can be given

Answer Key

1. D   2. D   3. A   4. A   5. C   6. B

Reference

Purandare CN, Suvarna Khadilkar. Menopause: Current Concepts: 2004 , Jaypee under auspices of FOGSI

Tibolone

◼ *Seema Sharma*

1. **State True or False**
   A. Tibolone is a STEAR hormone (selective tissue estrogenic activity regulator)
   B. Tibolone is a SERM (selective estrogen receptor modulator)
   C. Tibolone has no direct action on bone vagina and brain
   D. A and β hydroxy tibolone are the active metabolite
   E. It increases estradiol levels locally within the breast tissue
   F. It decreases estradiol levels within the breast tissue
   G. Tibolone causes selective activation of estrogen and progesterone receptors
   H. Tibolone causes selective activation of sulfatase and inhibition of sulfonyl transferase enzymes

2. **Following is True about tibolone:**
   A. It is a non-steroidal HRT
   B. It is a synthetic steroid
   C. It stimulates estrogen receptors at all sites
   D. It has no progestogenic property

3. **Tibolone has been used for the following indication except:**
   A. Prevention of postmenopausal osteoporosis
   B. Treatment of climacteric symptoms
   C. Treatment of postmenopausal osteoporosis
   D. Prevention of breast cancer

4. **The metabolites of tibolone include all except:**
   A. Delta 3-isomer
   B. Delta 4-isomer
   C. 3α-OH-tibolone
   D. 3β-OH-tibolone

5. **Metabolites α and β hydroxy tibolone have following action:**
   A. Estrogenic
   B. Progestogenic
   C. Androgenic
   D. All of the above

6. **delta 4-isomer has affinity for the following receptors:**
   A. Estrogen receptors
   B. Estrogen and progesterone receptors
   C. Progesterone and androgen receptors
   D. Estrogen and androgen receptors

7. **The effects of tibolone on the female genital tract include all except:**
   A. Estrogenic effect on vagina
   B. Estrogenic effect on uterus

C. Progestogenic effect on the uterus

D. Androgenic effect on genital tract

8. Following is true about tibolone's action on bones:
   A. It increase bone turnover
   B. It has no effect on bone resorption
   C. Its action is mediated via stimulation of ER
   D. Serum and urinary calcium levels are increased

9. The changes in lipid profile with tibolone therapy include:
   A. Increase in HDL cholesterol
   B. Increase in LDL cholesterol
   C. Decrease in LDL cholesterol
   D. Decrease in HDL cholesterol

10. Tibolone is preferred over estrogen progestogen therapy in postmenopausal women with the following conditions:
    A. Breast cancer
    B. Endometrial cancer
    C. Hypertriglyceridemia
    D. Vertebral fractures

11. The androgenic action of tibolone includes all except:
    A. Protection against breast cancer
    B. Lowering of SHBG
    C. Improvement in libido
    D. Reduction in vaginal dryness

12. The long-term therapy with tibolone increase the risk of:
    A. Endometrial cancer
    B. Breast cancer
    C. Venous thromboembolism
    D. Acne and hirsutism

13. The appropriate dose of tibolone in postmenopausal women is:
    A. 1.25 mg per day
    B. 2.5 mg twice a day
    C. 2.5 mg per day
    D. 5 mg per day

14. Tibolone's tissue-specific activity includes all except:
    A. Estrogenic effect on breasts

B. Estrogenic effect on bones

C. Estrogenic effect on vagina

D. Progestogenic effect on uterus

15. Tibolone's effect on lipid metabolism causes reduction in the following except:
    A. LDL cholesterol
    B. Lipoprotein A
    C. HDL cholesterol
    D. Triglycerides

16. Tibolone therapy is recommended for:
    A. Perimenopausal women
    B. Recently menopausal women
    C. Women who are at least one year postmenopausal
    D. Women who are at least 5 years postmenopausal

17. The effect of tibolone on breast tissues includes:
    A. Increase in breast density
    B. Decrease in cell proliferation
    C. Decrease in differentiation and apoptosis
    D. Increase in sulfatase activity

18. Tibolone supplements in postmenopausal women acts like:
    A. Oestrogen
    B. Progesterone
    C. Testosterone
    D. All of above

19. About tibolone, all are true except:
    A. Tibolone should not be used for cardiovascular protection
    B. Can increase risk of stroke, if it is used for more than 5–10 years after menopause
    C. Can be given in postmenopausal women with breast cancer
    D. Used to replace body's natural sex hormone in postmenopausal women

20. All of the following appear to decrease hot flushes in menopausal women except:
    A. Androgen

B. Raloxifene

C. Isoflavones

D. Tibolone

21. The elimination half-life of tibolone is approximately _____ hours:

A. 24

B. 30

C. 45

D. 60

22. Tibolone is a better option for post-menopausal women with diabetes mellitus.

A. True

B. False

Answer Key

1. State true or false		4. A	10. C	16. C	22. A
A True	E False	5. A	11. A	17. B	
B False	F True	6. C	12. D	18. D	
C True	G True	7. B	13. C	19. C	
D True	H False	8. C	14. A	20. B	
	2. B	9. D	15. A	21. C	
	3. D				

Explanations

1.	**C** True	Tibolone has no direct action on bone vagina and brain or any other tissues as it exerts its actions only through its metabolites which are active
	E False	Tibolone causes selective activation of sulfatase and inhibition of sulfotransferase
	F True	enzymes. Inhibition of sulfatase decreases conversion of estrone sulfatase to estrone
	H False	and thereby decreases estradiol production and also by inducing sulfotransferase brings about production of estradiol sulfate and estrone sulfate, hence reduces estradiol levels
15	**A**	Tibolone reduces levels of HDL, triglycerides and lipoprotein A but LDL levels are unaffected

Reference

Purandare CN, Suvarna Khadilkar, Menopause: Current Concepts: 2004, Jaypee under auspices of FOGSI

Selective Estrogen Receptor Modulator (SERM)

◘ *Suvarna Khadilkar*

Classify selective estrogen receptor modulators by generations: Mark the generation

I. *First generation*: Endometrial stimulation possible

II. *Second generation*: No endometrial stimulations, but precipitation of vasomotor symptoms

III. *Third generation*: No vasomotor symptoms

1. Lasofoxifene
2. Clomifene
3. Bazedoxifenes
4. Ospemifene
5. Raloxifene
6. Tamoxifene
7. Torimefene

True or False

8. Bazedoxifene in combination with estrogen is USFDA licenced in 2013 for prevention of postmenopausal posteoporosis.

9. Raloxifene is recommended for postmenopausal symptoms like hot flushes, and other vasomotor symptoms.

10. The most importanant side effect of raloxifene is thromboembolism.

11. Tamoxifene is useful in endometrial and breast cancer treatment.

12. Raloxifene is a:
    A. Steroid
    B. Benzothiophene derivative
    C. Drug which stimulates TAF2
    D. All of the above

13. Raloxifene:
    A. Stimulates bone formation
    B. Stimulates endometrial proliferation
    C. Prevents receptor negative breast cancer
    D. None of the above

14. Use of raloxifene:
    A. Is approved for prevention and treatment of osteoporosis
    B. Is approved only for treatment of osteoporosis
    C. Is approved for treatment of CA breast
    D. None of the above

15. More study involving 7705 postmenopausal women showed that:
    A. Reduction of risk of vertebral fracture by 30%
    B. Rise in BMD by 2–3% in spine and hip

C. Both A and B correct

D. None of the above

16. Raloxifene is a potent activator of transcription:

A. With ER β

B. With ER α

C. TAF2

D. All of the above

17. It is associated with all side effects except:

A. Increased risk of thromboembolism

B. Increased risk of hot flushes

C. Decreased HDL levels

D. Leg cramps

18. Raloxifene is to be used with caution with all of the following except:

A. Warfarin

B. Diazepam

C. Alendronate

D. Lidocaine

Answer Key

1. III	4. III	7. I	10. True	13. D	16. A
2. I	5. II	8. True	11. False	14. A	17. C
3. III	6. I	9. False	12. B	15. C	18. C

Reference

Purandare CN, Suvarna Khadilkar, Menopause: Current Concepts: 2004, Jaypee under auspices of FOGSI chapter 20.

Chapter 21

Alternate Therapy in Menopause

◨ *Shobhana Mohan Das*

1. Intestinal bacterial metablolism converts dietary daidzen to _____, a nonsteroidal estrogen.
   A. Glycone
   B. Genistein
   C. Cystein
   D. Equol

2. Cystein sulfoxide, (GPCS) that inhibits osteoclast activity is present in:
   A. Apple
   B. Soya beans
   C. Onion
   D. Flax seed

3. Isoflavones exist as glucosides and aglycones. Which is the enzyme that hydrolyses glucosides to aglycones:
   A. Glucosidase
   B. Hydroxylase
   C. Malonase
   D. None of the above

4. When soya beans are stored at room temperature for 3 years:
   A. Level of glucosides, increased, greatly followed by aglycones and malonylglucosides decreased
   B. Level of all isoflavones increased

   C. Level of glucosides decreased, but that of aglycones and malonylglucosides increased
   D. There was no change

5. What is the phytoestrogen commonly found in flax seed/linseed?
   A. Isoflavones
   B. Lignans
   C. Genistein
   D. Biochanin A

6. Phytoestrogens in general:
   A. Bind only to ER- Alfa
   B. Bind only to ER- Beta
   C. Have greater affinity to ER Alfa
   D. Have greater Affinity to ER- beta

7. A mixture of Cynanchum wilfordii, Phlomis umbrosa and Angelica gigas has been found in one study to reduce Kupperman's menopausal index in 3 months. This product is called.
   A. Phyto E
   B. Soy Iso
   C. Estro G
   D. Meno E

8. Yellow green colour of spinach comes from the presence of:
   A. Leutine and zeaxanthin
   B. β–cryptoxanthines and flavonoids

C. Glucosinolates and indoles

D. Anthocyanines and polyphenols

9. **Purple/red colour of berries/grapes come due to:**
   A. Leutine and zeaxanthin
   B. β-cryptoxanthines and flavonoids
   C. Glucosinolates and indoles
   D. Anthocyanines and polyphenols

10. **Orange/yellow colour of peaches, papaya and oranges come from:**
    A. Leutine and zeaxanthin.
    B. Alfa and β carotene
    C. Glucosinolates and indoles
    D. Anthocyanines and polyphenols

11. **Green colour of broccoli, cabbage and cauliflower comes from:**
    A. Leutine and zeaxanthin
    B. Alfa and β carotene
    C. Glucosinolates and indoles
    D. Anthocyanines and polyphenols

12. **Plant lignans are converted to mammalian lignans in the gut. Which of the following are mammalian lignans?**
    A. Secoisolariciresinol and matairesinol
    B. Enterodiol and enterolactone
    C. Secoisolariciresinol and enterodiol
    D. Matairesinol and enterolactone

13. **Grapes contain this element which is an estrogen enhancer:**
    A. Calcium
    B. Boron
    C. Iodine
    D. Selenium

14. **Which of the following statements is true?**
    Caffeine in coffee and tannin in tea can
    A. Cause more of calcium loss
    B. Improve vascular resistance
    C. Act as antioxidants
    D. Have anti-inflammatory properties

15. **Which of the following statements is true?**
    A. Curdling fresh soymilk with a coagulant produces tofu
    B. Soaking finely ground soybeans in water produces miso
    C. Ageing soya beans with grain-like rice for 1–3 years can make soymilk
    D. Fermenting uncooked soya beans and fried tofu can form natto a topping for rice

16. **This product was first reported in 1957 as a new phytoestrogen isolated from ladino clover, strawberry clover and alfalfa.**
    A. Lignan
    B. Isoflavon
    C. Coumestrol
    D. Diadzen

17. **Isolated isoflavones 165 mg/day at molecular level is approximately equivalent to:**
    A. 0.15 mg conjugated equine estrogen
    B. 0.3 mg conjugated equine estrogen
    C. 0.625 mg conjugated equine estrogen
    D. 1.25 mg conjugated equine estrogen

18. **Which of the following statements is false?**
    A. Soy feeding can suppress LH and FSH surge
    B. Soy feeding can decrease follicular phase estradiol
    C. Soy feeding increase follicular phase length
    D. Soy feeding can increase luteal phase length

19. **Which of the following statements are true?**
    In vitro studies have shown isoflavones to have antidiabetic properties, by
    1. Inhibiting intestinal brush border uptake of glucose
    2. Having glucosidase inhibitor action
    3. Demonstrating tyrosine kinase inhibitory properties

4. Multiple action on insulin release from pancreatic islet cells
  A. 1 and 2
  B. 2 and 3
  C. All are false
  D. All are true

20. Increased consumption of lettuce, spinach, herbal tea, and apples may:
  A. Protect against premenopausal breast cancer
  B. Increase the chance for breast cancer
  C. Can have no effect on the incidence of breast cancer

21. Proper absorption of isoflavones requires:
  A. Healthy bacterial flora
  B. Normal intestinal lining
  C. Adequate calcium
  D. Adequate acid secretion

22. For isoflavones to be effective genistein levels should be:
  A. 10 mmol / litre
  B. 25 mmol/ litre
  C. 50 mmol / litre
  D. 100 mmol/ litre

23. Phytoestrogens function by binding to _____receptor:
  A. ER-α only
  B. Er-β only
  C. Both A and B
  D. ER Delta

24. Isoflavones act through active forms such as:
  A. Genistin and daidzen
  B. Daidzen only
  C. Flavones
  D. Flavonoids

25. Isoflavones are basically _____ molecule.
  A. Fat-soluble
  B. Water soluble
  C. Acid soluble
  D. None of the above

26. Target tissue for isoflavones is/are:
  A. Reproductive tissue
  B. Skeletal tissue
  C. Cardiovascular tissue
  D. All of the above

27. Ideal dosage of isoflavones should be:
  A. 1–2 mg/kg per day
  B. 4 mg /kg per day
  C. 6 mg /kg per day
  D. 10 mg/kg per day

28. Mechanism of action of isoflavones is/are:
  A. Binding of estrogen receptor
  B. Modulation of sex steroid binding protein
  C. Inhibition of 5–α reductase
  D. All of the above

29. Soy provides isoflavones as:
  A. Biochanin A only
  B. Formonetin only
  C. Both A + B
  D. None of the above

Answer Key

1. D	6. C	11. C	16. C	21. A	26. D
2. C	7. C	12. B	17. B	22. B	27. A
3. A	8. A	13. B	18. D	23. C	28. D
4. A	9. D	14. A	19. D	24. A	29. C
5. B	10. B	15. A	20. A	25. A	

Explanations and References

2. **C.** A common vegetable with bone protective properties that is consumed worldwide is onion (*Allium cepe*). The aqueous residue after aqueous ethanol fractionation from dried onion bulb has been found to decrease bone reabsorption and to increase bone mineral content (BMC), trabecular thickness, and trabecular BMD in growing male rats.
    Reference: Jameela Banu, et al. Alternative therapies for the prevention and treatment of osteoporosis: Nutritional Reviews; 2012 Jan; 70(1):22–40.

3. **A.** Rekha CR, Vijayalakshmi G. International Journal of Food Sciences and Nutrition, March 2011; 62(2): 111–20.

4. **A.** Inge Lise Finn, et al. Nutrition and Cancer, 57(1), 1–10 Copyright C _ 2007, Lawrence Erlbaum Associates, Inc.

5. **B** Poulsen RC, et al. Soy phytoestrogens: Impact on postmenopausal bone loss and mechanisms of action: Nutrition Reviews Vol. 66(7): 359–74.

7. **C.** Phytother Res.2012 Apr, 26(4): 510–6.

12. **B.** Kurzer MS, et al. Dietary phytoestrogens:Annu. Rev. Nutr.1997.17:353–81.

16. **C.** Osoki AL, et al. Phytoestrogens: A Review of the Present State of Research Phytother. Res. 2003; (17) 845–69.

17. **B** Umland, et al. Phytoestrogens as HRT in Postmenopausal women: Pharmacotherapy 2000; 20(8)981–90.

18. **D** Annu. Rev. Nutr. 1997. 17:353–81.

19. **D** Cheng SY, et al. The Hypoglycemic Effects of Soy Isoflavones on Postmenopausal Women: Journal of Women's health,Volume 13, Number 10, 2004 © Mary Ann Liebert, Inc.

20. **A** Sanchez LT, et al. Food Sources of Phytoestrogens and Breast
    Cancer Risk in Mexican Women; Nutrition and Cancer, 37(2), 134–9.
    It has been suggested that phytoestrogens, which are hormone like compounds found in plant foods, might play a protective role in the etiology of breast cancer. These foods are also rich in the flavonoid quercetin. Quercetin inhibits the proliferation of human breast cancer cells *in vitro* and delays mammary tumorigenesis *in vivo*. Potential mechanisms for the anticarcinogenic effects of quercetin might include its capacity to bind with type II estrogen receptors and its potent antioxidant activity.

Case Scenarios:
Menopause Management

☐ *Suvarna Khadilkar*

CASE 1

- 44-year-old woman for health check
- Was asymptomatic, but now gets hot flushes
- Hypothyroid, on thyroxine since 12 years
- Sister had a hip fracture at age 54
- BMI 18
- Last period 6 months back.

Her dexa report shows following:

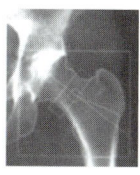
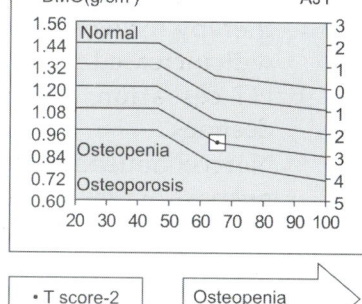
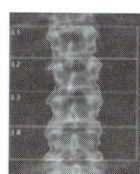

DMO(g/cm')		AJT
1.56 Normal		3
1.44		2
1.32		1
1.20		0
1.08		1
0.96		2
0.84 Osteopenia	⊡↔	3
0.72 Osteoporosis		4
0.60		5
20 30 40 50 60 70 80 90 100		

• T score-2 → Osteopenia

The result of DXA: T score-2

1. What would be the mode of management?
   A. No treatment
   B. Phytoestrogens
   C. Bisphosphonates
   D. Hormone therapy

2. If hormone therapy with estrogen and progesterone is opted, what would be ideal choice of regime?
   A. Continuous combined therapy
   B. Cyclic combined therapy
   C. Continuous sequential therapy
   D. Cyclic sequential therapy

CASE 2: Obese, 42-year-old perimeno-pausal woman seeks relief of menopausal symptoms, desires contraception, and needs control of bleeding which has been heavy since the past few months and has no medical problems.

3. What would be the next step in management of this case?
   A. Transvaginal ultrasonography pelvis
   B. Dilatation and curettage
   C. Hysteroscopy
   D. Hormone therapy

4. If hormonal therapy is chosen which would be the preferred option?
   A. Oral contraceptive pills
   B. Conjugated equine estrogens + medroxyprogesterone
   C. 17B estradiol + duphaston
   D. Conjugated equine estrogens+ Mirena

CASE 3
- 46 years old healthy women, para 2, breastfed
- Severe hot flushes, night sweats, insomnia, mood changes, loss of libido since 18 months
- LMP – 10 months ago
- H/O premenstrual breast pain
- Breast cyst aspirated 3 years ago
- Screening: Mammogram benign with dense breast
- After WHI previous reports refused hormone therapy, preferring non hormonal therapy for the past six months
- Unhappy with the relief has come back for consultation
- Close friend had a breast tumor
- She was afraid that her cyst would produce pain or neoplasm
- Although she did not want irregular bleeding she was willing to accept a regular predictable vaginal bleed

5. Would you offer her HT?
   A. Yes
   B. No

6. All of the following statements are True except:
   A. Hormonal therapy will cure her symptoms flushes, night sweats, bad sleep, mood changes and libido loss
   B. She is at a higher risk of having ca breast
   C. Her bone mineral density will improve with HT
   D. Cyclic sequential HT will be preferred regime for her

CASE 4
- Mrs D, 57-year-old woman consults you with a query on her HT
- She has been on cyclic EPT therapy for past 4 years after complete amenorrhea
- It was prescribed to her for management of VMS and vaginal dryness
- The therapy has been very effective with very few side effects
- She has now decided to discontinue with HT
- She wants to know the way forward

7. If she wants to stop the HT what would be your advise?
   A. Stop abruptly
   B. The dose and duration should be tapered
   C. She should be prescribed a phytoestrogens after stopping HT
   D. All of the above are correct
   E. Both A and B are correct

8. If she reconsiders her decision and wants to continue HT what would be your advice?
   A. She can continue for two more years
   B. She can continue for six more years
   C. She should continue smallest possible dose for shortest possible duration and review periodically
   D. She should shift to another drug regime

9. Which statement is not true regarding menopausal hormone therapy:
   A. HT is an appropriate first line therapy for women under age 60 with increased risk of fracture
   B. HT cessation, protective effect declines
   C. Not recommended after 60 for sole purpose of prevention of fractures
   D. Can be recommended after 60 years for treatment of osteoporosis

10. In case of surgical menopause:
    A. Routine HT is recommended for surgical menopause in postmenopausal women as primary prevention for chronic conditions
    B. Routine HT is recommended for surgical menopause in postmenopausal women as secondary prevention for chronic conditions
    C. HT should be considered in women less than the natural age of

menopause who have undergone surgical menopause

D. HT is not recommended in surgical menopause for managing

menopausal symptoms if they are beyond the natural age of menopause

Answer Key

1. D	3. A	5. A	7. E	9. D
2. D	4. D	6. B	8. C	10. C

Chapter

23

Metabolic Syndrome and Obesity

◨ *Neelam Aggarwal*

1. Which of the following criteria for metabolic syndrome varies by race/ethnicity?
   A. Hypertension
   B. Fasting plasma glucose levels
   C. Waist circumference
   D. HDL-C levels

2. Which of the following is correct for metabolic syndrome?
   A. HDL-C < 50 mg/dL and blood pressure ≥ 120/75 mm Hg
   B. HDL-C < 50 mg/dL and blood pressure ≥ 130/85 mm Hg
   C. HDL-C < 35 mg/dL and blood pressure ≥ 135/85 mm Hg
   D. HDL-C < 30 mg/dL and blood pressure ≥ 140/90 mm Hg

3. Which of the following lifestyle changes is most beneficial for reduced risk of coronary heart disease?
   A. Switching to low fat milk
   B. Exercising on a daily basis
   C. Taking iron and multivitamin supplement
   D. Reducing the working hours

4. Which of the following is not part of the 'metabolic syndrome'?
   A. High triglycerides
   B. Blood pressure 130/80 mm Hg
   C. Obesity
   D. Low HDL

5. The mechanism of action of Orlistat is:
   A. Promotes satiety
   B. Inhibits appetite center
   C. Increases BMR
   D. Inhibits gastric and pancreatic lipases

6. All of the following are cause of secondary obesity except:
   A. Hypothyroidism
   B. Insulinoma
   C. Diabetes mellitus
   D. Cushing's syndrome

7. Regarding effect of HRT on weight gain, which is true:
   A. Increases the risk of weight gain
   B. Increases the risk of android obesity
   C. Deteriorates HbA1c levels
   D. Improves insulin resistance

8. What is the range of BMI for overweight?
   A. 15–18.5%
   B. 18.5–25%
   C. 25–29.9%
   D. > 30%

9. All are risk factors for metabolic syndrome except:
   A. Insulin resistance
   B. Hypertension
   C. Dyslipidemia
   D. Low levels of CRP

10. The first line treatment of metabolic syndrome is:
    A. Weight loss medications
    B. Weight loss
    C. Insulin sensitizers
    D. Lifestyle measures

11. Which of the following is bad:
    A. Subcutaneous fat
    B. Visceral fat
    C. Fat around your thighs
    D. Fat in the breast tissue

12. Which of the following is not true regarding visceral fat:
    A. It is inside abdomen surrounding the organs
    B. Is linked to an increase in insulin resistance
    C. This is more dangerous than subcutaneous fat
    D. It is metabolically less active

13. Obesity in perimenopausal women leads to:
    A. Increased risk of leiomyosarcoma
    B. Increased risk of insulin resistance
    C. Deteriorates hypothyroidism
    D. Improves insulin resistance

14. BMI is expressed as:
    A. Weight (kg)/height (m^2)
    B. Weight (lb)/height (m^2)
    C. Height (m)/weight (kg)
    D. Weight (kg)/height m^2)

15. What is the range of BMI for ideal weight?
    A. 15–18.5%
    B. 18.5–25%
    C. 25–29.9%
    D. > 30%

16. Which of the following is true about fat redistribution in perimenopausal and menopausal women?
    A. From subcutaneous to visceral fat
    B. From visceral to subcutaneous fat
    C. Development of lower obesity
    D. Pear-shaped obesity

17. Which of the following is not associated with obesity?
    A. Insulin resistance
    B. Cardiovascular diseases
    C. Musculoskeletal diseases
    D. Osteoporosis

18. Not true about diagnosis of metabolic syndrome:
    A. Abdominal obesity defined as > 35 inches in females
    B. BP > 130/85
    C. S. Triglycerides < 150 mg/dL
    D. Plasma glucose > 110 mg/dL

19. Almost 75% of patients with type–2 diabetes or impaired glucose tolerance have the metabolic syndrome.
    A. True
    B. False

Answer Key

1. C	5. D	9. D	13. B	17. D
2. B	6. C	10. D	14. A	18. C
3. B	7. D	11. B	15. A	19. A
4. B	8. C	12. D	16. A	

Explanations

1. **C** According to guidelines from the National Heart, Lung, and Blood Institute (NHLBI) and the American Heart Association (AHA), metabolic syndrome is diagnosed when a patient has at least 3 of the following 5 conditions:
    (a) Fasting glucose ≥ 100 mg/dL (or receiving drug therapy for hyperglycemia)
    (b) Blood pressure ≥ 130/85 mm Hg (or receiving drug therapy for hypertension)
    (c) Triglycerides ≥ 150 mg/dL (or receiving drug therapy for hypertriglyceridemia)
    (d) HDL-C < 40 mg/dL in men or < 50 mg/dL in women (or receiving drug therapy for reduced HDL-C)
    (e) Waist circumference ≥ 102 cm (40 in) in men or ≥ 88 cm (35 in) in women; if Asian American, ≥ 90 cm (35 in) in men or ≥ 80 cm (32 in) in women.

5. **D** This is the only FDA approved drug for use in weight loss.

11. **B** Visceral fat is more active metabolically and has a negative impact.

14. **A** The BMI is universally expressed in kg/m², resulting from mass in kilograms and height in metres. If pounds and inches are used, a conversion factor of 703 (kg/m²)/(lb/in²) must be applied.

15. **A** BMI provides a simple numeric measure of a person's thickness or thinness, to discuss weight problems more objectively. The current value recommendations are as follow:
    - BMI from 18.5 up to 25 kg/m² may indicate optimal weight
    - BMI lower than 18.5 suggests the person is underweight
    - Number from 25 up to 30 may indicate the person is overweight
    - A number from 30 upwards suggests the person is obese.

16. **A** The perimenopausal period is associated with a rapid increase in fat mass with redistribution from subcutaneous to visceral sites leading to the development of android obesity (apple shape in place of pear).

17 **D** Androgens are converted to oestrogen in fatty tissue, so obesity is protective.

Comorbidities at Menopause

◾ *Jyothi Unni*

1. Which of the following blood tests is most indicative of cardiac damage?
   - A. Lactate dehydrogenase
   - B. Troponin T
   - C. Creatinine kinase
   - D. Fibrin degradation products

2. What is the first thing to do in a patient with signs and symptoms of coronary artery disease?
   - A. Increase oxygenation
   - B. Allay anxiety
   - C. Give sublingual nitroglycerin
   - D. Give digoxin

3. 51 years old, c/o hot flushes and night sweats. Amenorrhoea of 1 year. BMI 30, BP 150/100. Which is the best treatment option?
   - A. Raloxifene
   - B. Oral estrogen
   - C. Tibolone
   - D. Transdermal estrogen

4. The effect of oral estrogen on the lipid profile is true in all statements except:
   - A. Decreases triglycerides
   - B. Increases HDL cholesterol
   - C. Decreases LDL cholesterol
   - D. Decreases total cholesterol

5. 47 years old, asymptomatic woman. BMI: 18 hypothyroid on thyroxine for 15 years. What is her main risk?
   - A. Coronary artery disease
   - B. Cerebrovascular accident
   - C. Osteoporosis
   - D. Alzheimer's disease

6. 45 years old with a history of radical mastectomy 7 years ago for Ca breast, complains of vaginal dryness and dyspareunia. What would you offer?
   - A. Clonidine
   - B. Vaginal estrogen
   - C. Tibolone
   - D. Phytoesrogen

7. 60 years old, with history of CABG done 2 years ago. Undergone hysterectomy for fibroids 12 years ago. Complains of night sweats, mood swings, insomnia. What treatment would you offer her?
   - A. Estrogen + progesterone
   - B. Venlaflaxine
   - C. Estrogen
   - D. Evening primrose oil

8. A postmenopausal woman who is overweight, hypertensive and diabetic presents with per vaginum

bleeding. Following diagnosis is more likely:

A. Endometrial cancer
B. DUB
C. Senile endometritis
D. Ca cervix

9. Estrogen has a protective effect on cardiovascular health by all the following except:

A. Beneficial effect on lipids and lipoproteins
B. Dilatation of vascular smooth muscles
C. Antioxidant
D. Increase in platelet aggregation

10. All the following are components of Alzheimer's disease except:

A. Amnesia (memory)
B. Agnosia (recognition)
C. Ataxia (balance)
D. Aphasia (spoken language)

Answers Key

1. B	3. D	5. C	7. B	9. D
2. A	4. A	6. B	8. A	10. C

Chapter

25

Thyroid Disorders at Perimenopause

◉ *Suvarna Khadilkar and Seema sharma*

1. Thyroid hormones affect the reproductive function both directly and indirectly through which of the following mechanisms:
   A. Increase the synthesis of sex hormone binding globulin (SHBG)
   B. Altered testosterone and androstenedione levels
   C. Reduce the clearance of estradiol and androgens
   D. Increase the conversion of androgens to estrone.
   E. All of the above

2. Subclinical hypothyroidism is said to be present:
   A. TSH is low and free T3/T4 is normal
   B. TSH is high and free T3/T4 is normal
   C. TSH is high and free T3/T4 is high
   D. None of the above

3. Incidence of thyroid disease in postmenopausal women is:
   A. Clinical thyroid disease: 2.4%
   B. Subclinical thyroid disease: 23.2%
   C. 73.8% are hypothyroid and 26.2% are hyperthyroid amongst subclinical thyroid disease
   D. All of the above are correct

4. All of the following symptoms of thyroid dysfunction mimic menopause except:
   A. Fatigue
   B. Poor memory
   C. Lethargy, depression, mood swings
   D. Change in libido/sex drive
   E. Weight gain
   F. Hair loss changes in hair texture
   G. Sleep disturbances
   H. Irregular or missed menstrual periods
   I. Palpitations

5. True or false:
   A. Primary hypothyroidism is caused most commonly by autoimmune thyroiditis
   B. Secondary hypothyroidism occurs due to decreased TSH secretion by pituitary
   C. Hypothyroidism caused by various drugs is termed tertiary hypothyroidism
   D. Chemotherapeutic agents ipilimumab, bexarotene, sunitinib (tyrosine kinase inhibitors) can cause hypothyroidism

E. Consumptive hypothyroidism occurs as a paraneoplastic condition

6. Following are recommended for treatment of hypothyroidism:
   A. Levothyroxine
   B. Desiccated thyroid extract
   C. Isolated T3 hormone replacement
   D. A and B
   E. A and C

7. What are the most commonly followed cut offs for TSH levels internationally?
   A. .2–2.5 mIU/L
   B. .4–4.5 mIU/L
   C. .1–10 mIU/L
   D. None of the above

8. When do patients with high TSH require treatment?
   A. If TSH is more than 10
   B. If TSH is between 5–10 and having symptoms
   C. If TSH is between 5–10 and anti TPO antibodies test is positive
   D. If TSH is more than 5 and having evidence of atherosclerotic heart disease
   E. All of the above

9. Which of the following is not a feature of malignant thyroid nodule by ultrasound?
   A. Microcalcifications
   B. Marked hypoechogenicity
   C. Irregular or microlobulated margin
   D. Vascularity surrounding the nodule on Doppler
   E. Longitudinal dimension larger than the cross-sectional dimension

10. Following is not true about menopausal hormone therapy and the thyroid disease:
    A. MHT in women with hypothyroidism does not alter free thyroxine and TSH levels
    B. There is increased need for thyroxine while on MHT
    C. TSH levels are stabilized by 12 weeks after the beginning of therapy
    D. Increased binding of thyroxine to elevated thyroxine-binding globulin leads to elevated TSH

11. All of the following are true about thyroid dysfunction at menopause except:
    A. Their incidence is 15–20 times higher in women than in men
    B. Prevalence of most thyroid diseases decreases at menopause
    C. Diagnosis of thyroid disease is difficult at menopause
    D. Low thyroid function relates to dyslipidemia

12. Thyroid cancer and its treatment relate to worse outcome in postmenopausal women than in the young population.
    A. True
    B. False

13. Thyroid dysfunction increases cardiovascular risk and cardiovascular and general mortality, and hyperthyroidism leads to increased risk of osteoporotic fractures in postmenopausal women.
    A. True
    B. False

14. Which of the following is true about thyroid cancer?
    A. Incidence of differentiated thyroid cancer decreases in population over 55 years old
    B. Incidence of anaplastic thyroid cancer decreases in those aged over 65 years
    C. Higher prevalence of thyroid lymphoma and sarcoma is noted in younger population
    D. The genetic background of papillary carcinoma differs according to the age

15. Most important preoperative diagnostic procedure in postmenopausal women with thyroid cancer is:
A. Fine-needle aspiration biopsy
B. Ultrasonography
C. CT-scan
D. X-ray

Answer Key

1. E	5. A True	E True	9. D	13. A
2. B	B True	6. A	10. A	14. D
3. D	C False	7. B	11. B	15. A
4. E	D True	8. E	12. A	

Explanation and Reference

3. **D** Schindler AE1.Thyroid function and Postmenopause. Gynecol Endocrinol. 2003 Feb; 17(1):79–85. Germany

14 **D** In 40–60% of older patients activating BRAF mutation is observed, while in 50% of children and 25% of adults < 45 years old RET/PTC rearrangement is the major genetic event leading to carcinogenesis.

Endocrinopathies at Perimenopause

▣ *Suvarna Khadilkar*

1. As per WHO estimates all of the following are true about burden of diabetes in India except:
   A. Diabetes type 2 incidence in 2007 was 30%
   B. Diabetes type 2 incidence in India as in 2010 was 51%
   C. Men suffer from diabetes mellitus type 2 more than women
   D. Diabetes type 2 incidence in India by 2030 is expected to be 80%

2. Following facts about HbA1c test are true except:
   A. It has a diagnostic value
   B. It has a prognostic value
   C. It can replace fasting blood sugar estimation in work-up of a diabetis mellitus
   D. It is an indicator of chronic glycemic control

3. Thyroid related osteoporosis: State true or false:
   A. Long-term hypothyroidism leads to osteoporosis
   B. Long-term treatment with levo-thyroxine leads to osteoporosis
   C. Hyperthyroidism leads to osteoporosis
   D. Antithyroid medication leads to osteoporosis

4. Diabetes in menopausal age group:
   A. Presence of type 2 diabetes mellitus in women reverses the cardiovascular protective effects of endogenous estrogens before menopause
   B. Hyperglycemia and insulin resistance/hyperinsulinemia negate 'estrogen protection' in premenopausal diabetic women
   C. None of the above
   D. Both A and B are correct

5. Dose of injection teriparatide (rPTH) for postmenopausal women with severe osteoporosis at high-risk of fractures is:
   A. 20 micrograms subcutaneously daily maximum for two years
   B. 50 micrograms weekly for 6 months
   C. 75 micrograms once a month for twelve months
   D. None of the above

Answer Key

1. C	3. A False	C True	4. D
2. C	B True	D False	5. A

Carcinoma Breast

◙ *Kawita Bapat*

1. Which of the following are possible symptoms of breast cancer?
   A. A change in the size or shape of the breast
   B. Nipple discharge or tenderness
   C. Orange peel appearance of the breast
   D. All of the above

2. Which of the following are true of breast cancer?
   A. Life time risk for a woman developing breast cancer is one in nine
   B. For most women a specific cause of their breast cancer is known
   C. Prognosis is worse for affluent women
   D. Incidence of breast cancer is decreasing

3. The following statements regarding screening for breast cancer are correct.
   A. Mammography should be offered to all women between the ages of 50 and 75 years
   B. Studies have shown an approximate 30% reduction in mortality with screening using mammography

C. Most radiographically suspicious lesions are subsequently confirmed as malignant
   D. Mammography is less sensitive in postmenopausal women

4. Which of the following is not indicated when a patient first presents with a breast lump?
   A. Fine needle aspiration (FNA)
   B. Chest X-ray
   C. Examination of axillary lymph nodes
   D. Examination of breasts with patient supine

5. Which of the following are good prognostic factors in breast cancer?
   A. Estrogen receptor positivity
   B. Grade III tumour
   C. HER 2 receptor overexpression
   D. Lymph node involvement

6. Which of the following statements is true regarding adjuvant treatment for early breast cancer?
   A. Radiotherapy is indicated after breast conserving surgery only if > 4 nodes positive or tumour close to the resection margin
   B. Aromatase inhibitors are replacing tamoxifen in premenopausal

women due to better outcomes and greater tolerability

C. Combination chemotherapy reduces recurrence and improves survival in selected patient groups

D. No survival benefit has been demonstrated with use of trastuzumab (herceptin) in the adjuvant setting

7. Which statement is true for treatment of metastatic breast cancer…
   A. Chemotherapy is superior to endocrine therapy
   B. Bisphosphonates are used to control hypocalcaemia
   C. Responses to endocrine therapy tend to occur within 2 months of starting treatment
   D. Trastuzumab (herceptin) in combination with chemotherapy improves survival in patients who have tumours that overexpress her 2

8. Which of the following statements is true of breast cancer treatment?
   A. Mastectomy is superior to breast conservation surgery
   B. Chemotherapy can be used safely in the first trimester of pregnancy
   C. Radiotherapy should be given to all male breast cancer patients after mastectomy
   D. Paget's disease of the nipple should be treated with wide local excision

9. Which of the following statements is true of palliative treatment of metastatic breast cancer?
   A. Hypercalcaemia should be treated with increased oral fluids and oral bisphosphonates
   B. Increased back pain and 'weak legs' requires prompt investigation
   C. Bisphosphonates are used in treatment of liver metastases
   D. Neuropathic pain usually responds quickly to opioid analgesics

10. Which of the following is a rare site of breast cancer metastases?
    A. Brain
    B. Kidney
    C. Liver
    D. Bone

11. All of the following trials on hormone therapy and menopause showed increase incidence of breast carcinoma except:
    A. WHI estrogen and progesterone trial
    B. Million women study
    C. HERS study
    D. WHI estrogen only trial

12. Liberate trial gave a significant conclusion. Pick out the correct one:
    A. Tibolone is safe in breast cancer survivors
    B. Tibolone should not be used as an option for menopausal symptoms as it causes breast cancer
    C. Tibolone should not be used in women with past history of cancer as it leads to recurrence of the carcinoma breast
    D. None of the above

13. How many times a month should a woman perform a self-exam?
    A. Once a month
    B. Twice every quarter
    C. Once a year
    D. Three times per year

14. What steps should you do in a routine breast self-exam?
    A. Look at breasts' size, shape, colour and discharge in the mirror
    B. Raise arms overhead and check for any changes in your breasts
    C. Lie down and feel each breast in circular motion; left hand to right breast, and right hand to left breast
    D. Check breasts while standing up or sitting down, even if in the shower
    E. All of the above

15. How should one perform a self-breast examination?
    A. Lightly touching the breast with one finger in no particular motion
    B. Use finger pads of your three middle fingers move the pads of your fingers in little circles, about the size of a dime. Start from your arm pit move down the bra line
    C. Moving fingers from top to bottom and side to side of each breast
    D. Use whole hand and lightly squeeze each breast

16. What other symptoms should women look for while checking her breasts for lumps?
    A. Nipple tenderness and/or if the nipple has turned inward or become inverted
    B. Change in shape or size of breast, with any unexplained shrinking of the breast
    C. Redness, swelling, enlarged pores or a scaly texture (similar to orange peel) on skin of breast, nipple and/or areola
    D. Discharge from nipple (clear, milky, bloody)
    E. All of the above

17. What are some other ways to reduce the risk of breast cancer besides routine self-exams?
    A. Maintaining a healthy weight
    B. Have clinical breast exams starting at age 20 and mammograms starting at age 40
    C. Breastfeeding, if possible, after giving birth
    D. Cutting down use of menopausal hormone therapy
    E. All of the above

18. The greatest risk of breast cancer occurs at what age?
    A. Under 30
    B. 30–49
    C. 50 and over
    D. Although all women are at risk

19. Most women diagnosed with breast cancer have:
    A. Family history of the disease
    B. Lumpy breast tissue
    C. High stress levels
    D. None of the above

20. Which of these has been proven to increase breast cancer risk?
    A. Cell phones
    B. Breast implants
    C. Antiperspirants
    D. None of the above

21. Which of the following diseases is associated with highest mortality rates for women?
    A. Colon cancer
    B. Breast cancer
    C. Lung cancer
    D. Heart disease

22. All are potential risk factors for carcinoma breast except:
    A. History of breast cancer in mother or sister, especially while premenopausal
    B. Diet high in vegetables and fruits
    C. Exposure to intense radiation
    D. Long-term use (> 5 years) of estrogen plus progestogen

Answer Key

1. D	5. C	9. B	13. A	17. E	21. D
2. A	6. C	10. B	14. E	18. C	22. B
3. A	7. D	11. D	15. B	19. D	
4. B	8. D	12. C	16. E	20. D	

Menopause and Cancer

◉ *Punit Bhojani*

1. The commonest malignancy in women irrespective of age is:
   A. Carcinoma cervix
   B. Carcinoma breast
   C. Carcinoma esophagus
   D. Carcinoma endometrium

2. Staging of endometrial carcinomas is:
   A. Surgical
   B. Clinical
   C. Surgical + clinical
   D. None of the above

3. Staging of cervical carcinoma is:
   A. Surgical
   B. Radiological
   C. Clinical
   D. Clinical + surgical

4. Surgical treatment alone for cervical carcinomas is advocated in all of the following except:
   A. Stage 1a
   B. Stage 1b
   C. Stage 2a
   D. Stage 2b

5. Tamoxifen has _____ effect on breast tissue.
   A. Estrogen agonist
   B. Estrogen antagonist
   C. Estrogen agonist + antagonist
   D. None of the above

6. Raloxifene has _____ effect on endometrial tissue
   A. Estrogen antagonist
   B. Estrogen agonist
   C. Progestogenic
   D. Androgenic

7. Tibolone has all of the following properties except:
   A. Estrogenic
   B. Progestogenic
   C. Androgenic
   D. Thrombogenic

Answer Key

1. B	3. C	5. B	7. D
2. A	4. D	6. A	

Reference

Purandare CN, Suvarna Khadilkar. Menopause: Current Concepts: 2004, Jaypee under auspices of FOGSI Chapter 28.

Chapter
29

Cancer Cervix

◾ *Punit Bhojani*

1. Risk factors for cancer cervix (Ca cervix) are all except:
   A. HPV infection
   B. Nulliparity
   C. Polygamy
   D. Smoking

2. Most common HPV associated with CA cervix is:
   A. HPV 31
   B. HPV 16
   C. HPV 18
   D. HPV 45

3. CIN 1 will progress to cancer in __% cases.
   A. 5
   B. 10
   C. < 1
   D. 20

4. As per ACOG guidelines, women aged 23 years should have:
   A. PAP test every 5 years
   B. PAP test every 3 years
   C. No need for PAP test
   D. PAP test and HPV testing every 2 years

5. Patient can stop cervical cancer screening after the age of ___ years
   A. 45
   B. 55

   C. 65
   D. 75

6. Most common abnormal PAP test is:
   A. HSIL
   B. LSIL
   C. ASCUS
   D. ASC-H

7. Fixative for PAP smear is:
   A. Normal saline
   B. Formaldehyde
   C. Alcohol and ether
   D. 100% alcohol

8. Stage lb cervical cancer is diagnosed in a young woman. Assuming that the cancer is confined to the cervix and that intraoperative biopsies are negative which of the following structures can be conserved during radical hysterectomy for carcinoma cervix stage Ib?
   A. Uterosacral and uterovesical ligaments
   B. Pelvic nodes
   C. The entire parametrium on both sides of the cervix
   D. Both ovaries

9. Point B in the treatment of carcinoma cervix receives the following dose of radiation:

A. 7000 cGy
B. 6000 cGy
C. 5000 cGy
D. 10,000 cGy

10. A 50-year-old woman is diagnosed with cervical cancer. Which lymph node group would be the first to be involved in metastatic spread of this disease beyond the cervix and uterus?
A. Internal iliac nodes
B. Obturator nodes
C. External iliac nodes
D. Paracervical nodes

11. What is the cell of origin in most cases of Ca cervix?
A. Tall columnar cell
B. Squamous cell
C. Spindle cell
D. None of the above

12. Therapeutic conization is indicated in:
A. Microinvasive carcinoma cervix stage 1a1
B. CIN III
C. Unsatisfactory colposcopy with cervical dysplasia
D. Cervical metaplasia

13. A 55-year-old lady presenting to outpatient department with post-menopausal bleeding for 3 months has a 1 × 1 cm nodule on the anterior lip of cervix. The most appropriate investigation to be done subsequently is:
A. Pap smear
B. Punch biopsy
C. Endocervical curettage
D. Colposcopy

14. Radioisotope used in Ca cervix brachytherapy:
A. Cobalt
B. Iridium
C. Cesium
D. Any of the above

15. Wertheim's hysterectomy is done for:
A. IA1 cervical cancer
B. Selected cases of stage Ib

C. Germ cell ovarian cancer
D. All of the above

16. A stage 1A2 cervical cancer is detected at 26 weeks of pregnancy. Next line of management is:
A. LSCS followed by extrafascial hysterectomy at 28 weeks
B. Immediate CTRT
C. Classical cesarean section followed by Wertheim's hysterectomy at 30–32 weeks
D. MTP

17. Which proteins of HPV play a role in pathogenesis of cervical cancer?
A. E3, E4
B. E5, E6
C. E6, E7
D. E8, E10

18. Gardasil vaccine is for:
A. HPV 16, 18
B. HSV
C. HPV 6, 11, 16, 18
D. Hepatitis B

19. A 35-year-old lady has undergone radical hysterectomy for Ca cervix. Histopathology shows stage IBI with outer one-third of cervix and lower uterine segment involvement. No LVSI and tumor < 2 cm next line of management is:
A. Follow-up
B. Chemoradiation
C. Chemotherapy
D. Radiation

20. A patient presents with Ca cervix with stage IIIb; treatment of choice is:
A. Chemotherapy
B. Intracavitatory brachytherapy followed by external beam radiotherapy
C. Wertheim's hysterectomy
D. Chemoradiation

21. All are features of dysplastic cells except:
    A. Nuclear enlargement with variation in shape and size
    B. Hyperchromasia—increased intensity of staining
    C. Irregular chromatin distribution with clumping
    D. Mitotic figures and visible nuclei
    E. Inclusion bodies

22. All are true regarding HPV and cervical cancer except:
    A. Globally, currently available vaccines are bivalent, quadrivalent and nanovalent
    B. HPV vaccines can effectively prevent development of cervical cancer
    C. HPV vaccines should not be given to girls below 14 years
    D. None of the above

23. Following are the modalities of treatment of CIN except:
    A. Radical hysterectomy
    B. Cryotherapy
    C. LEEP (loop electrosurgical excision procedure)
    D. Conization

24. A 48 years old woman underwent routine pap smear, the most common finding is:
    A. Cells of deep layers with large nucleus
    B. Tadpole like cells
    C. Wafer like cells with pyknotic nucleus
    D. Clue cells

25. The most frequent gynecological cancer in India is:
    A. Cervical
    B. Endometrial
    C. Ovarian
    D. Vulvar

26. Recommendations by ACOG for cervical cytology, 2003: state true or false.
    A. Annual cervical cytology screening should begin three years after initiation of sexual intercourse no later than 21 years of age
    B. Women 30 years and older who have had three consecutive test results negative for intraepithelial lesions and malignancy may be screened every two to three years for rest of the life
    C. After age of 60 screening can be stopped if last three consecutive smears were negative
    D. Women infected with human immunodeficiency virus, immunosuppressed, women and diethylstilbestrol exposure *in utero* require 6 monthly screening
    E. That annual examinations, including pelvic examination, may not be necessary if regular cervical cytology screening is done
    F. Women who have had a total hysterectomy for benign indications and have no history of high-grade cervical intraepithelial neoplasia (CIN) should continue routine screening
    G. Women who have had a total hysterectomy and have a history of CIN 2 or 3, or in whom a negative history cannot be documented, should continue to be screened annually until three consecutive satisfactory negative vaginal cytology results are obtained

Answer Key

1. B	7. C	13. B	19. A	25. A	F. False
2. B	8. D	14. D	20. D	26. A. True	G. True
3. C	9. C	15. B	21. E	B. False	
4. B	10. D	16. C	22. C	C. True	
5. C	11. B	17. C	23. A	D. True	
6. C	12. A	18. C	24. A	E. False	

Explanations

1. **B** Risk factors for CA cervix:
   - Young age at first intercourse (<16 years)
   - Multiple sexual partners
   - Cigarette smoking
   - Race
   - High parity
   - Low socioeconomic status
   - Human papillomavirus (HPV) infection (main cause)
   - HIV
   - Immunosuppression

2. **B** HPV–16 is the most common HPV seen in invasive Ca and CIN 2/3 and is found in 50% cases.
   - HPV–16 is not very specific and is also the most common HPV type in women with normal cytology.
   - HPV–18 is more specific than HPV–16 for invasive tumors.

3. **C**

Cervical Epithelium	CIN I	CIN II	CIN III/CIS
Regression to normal (%)	60	40	30
Persistence (%)	30	35	50
Progression to CIN III/CIS (%)	10	20	–
Progression to invasion (%)	<1	5	20

4. **B**

6. **C** The different types of abnormal Pap test results:
   - Atypical squamous cells of undetermined significance (ASC-US)—ASC-US means that changes in the cervical cells have been found. The changes are almost always a sign of an HPV infection. ASC-US is the most common abnormal Pap test result.
   - Low-grade squamous intraepithelial lesion (LSIL)—LSIL means that the cervical cells show changes that are mildly abnormal. LSIL usually is caused by an HPV infection that often goes away on its own.
   - High-grade squamous intraepithelial lesion (HSIL)—HSIL suggests more serious changes in the cervix than LSIL. It is more likely than LSIL to be associated with precancer and cancer.
   - Atypical squamous cells, cannot exclude HSIL (ASC-H)—ASC-H means that changes in the cervical cells have been found that raise concern for the presence of HSIL.
   - Atypical glandular cells (AGC)—Glandular cells are another type of cell that make-up the thin layer of tissue that covers the inner canal of the cervix. Glandular cells also are present inside the uterus. An AGC result means that changes have been found in glandular cells that raise concern for the presence of precancer or cancer.

7. **C** Fixative for PAP smear is 95% ethyl alcohol and ether.

8. **D** (Both ovaries) Radical hysterectomy is most often used as a primary treatment for early cervical cancer (stage 1A2, 1B, and IIA), and occasionally as a primary treatment for uterine cancer. In either case, there must be no evidence of spread beyond the operative field, as suggested by negative intraoperative frozen-section biopsies. The procedure involves excision of the

uterus, the upper third of the vagina, the uterosacral and uterovesical ligaments, and all of the parametrium, and pelvic node dissection including the ureteral, obturator, hypogastric, and iliac nodes. Radical hysterectomy, thus, attempts to preserve the bladder, rectum, and ureters while excising as much as possible of the remaining tissue around the cervix that might be involved in microscopic spread of the disease. Ovarian metastases from cervical cancer are extremely rare. Preservation of the ovaries is generally acceptable, particularly in younger women.

10. **D** (Paracervical nodes) The main routes of spread of cervical cancer include vaginal mucosa, myometrium, paracervical lymphatics, and direct extension into the parametrium. The prevalence of lymph node disease correlates with the stage of malignancy. Primary node groups involved in the spread of cervical cancer include the paracervical (sentinel node), parametrial, obturator, hypogastric, external iliac, and sacral nodes, essentially in that order. Less commonly, there is involvement in the common iliac, inguinal, and para-aortic nodes.

12. **A** (Microinvasive carcinoma cervix stage 1a1) Stage 1A of Ca cervix is microinvasive. It is divided into 1A1 and 1A2.

   In stage 1A1, there is no lymph node involvement. Therapeutic conization is the surgery of choice for stage 1A1 in young patients who are desirous of future childbearing. If the patient is old or family is complete, then this stage is treated by simple hysterectomy.

   Option b = LEEP/LLETZ in young patients who are desirous of future childbearing. If the patient is old or family is complete, then this is treated by simple hysterectomy

   Option c = diagnostic conization.

   Option d = no treatment is required.

16. **C** (Classical cesarean section followed by Wertheim's hysterectomy at 30–32 weeks)

17. **C** (E6, E7) The initial event in cervical dysplasia and carcinogenesis is likely to be infection with HPV. The mechanism by which HPV affects cellular growth and differentiation is by interactions of viral E6 and E7 proteins with p53 and Rb resulting in gene activation.

19. **A** (Follow-up) Postoperative CTRT to the pelvis decreases the risk of local recurrence in patients with high-risk factors, such as:

   1. Positive pelvic nodes

   2. Positive surgical margins

   3. Residual parametrial disease

   If these were present, then the answer would be chemoradiation. As these are not present, only follow-up of the patient is required.

20. **D** Chemoradiation

   Stage-wise treatment for Ca cervix

   - All stages (I–IV) are radiosensitive.
   - Stages of Ca cervix that are operable (radical/Wertheim's hysterectomy) are 1A2, IB, and IIA.
   - Stages IIB-IV are not operable and have to be treated with RT only (brachy- and teletherapy)
   - Cisplatin is given before RT as a radiosensitizer.

Chapter 30

Endometrial Cancer

◾ Punit Bhojani

1. All are risk factors for Ca endometrium except:
   A. Late menopause
   B. Tamoxifen
   C. Multiparity
   D. Chronic Anovulation

2. Simple hyperplasia will progress to Ca endometrium in _____ % cases.
   A. 1
   B. 5
   C. 10
   D. 15

3. Corpus cancer syndrome includes all except:
   A. Obesity
   B. Hypertension
   C. Diabetes mellitus
   D. Atypical endometrial hyperplasia

4. A patient is receiving external beam radiation for the treatment of metastatic endometrial cancer. The treatment field includes the entire pelvis. Which of the following tissues within this radiation field is the most radiosensitive?
   A. Vagina
   B. Ovary
   C. Rectovaginal septum
   D. Bladder

5. Most common cause of post-menopausal uterine bleeding is:
   A. Endometrial atrophy
   B. Hormone replacement therapy
   C. Endometrial hyperplasia
   D. Endometrial Ca

6. Average age for Ca endometrium is:
   A. 35–45 years
   B. 45–50 years
   C. 60–70 years
   D. 75–80 years

7. Most common variety of Ca endometrium is:
   A. Adenocarcinoma
   B. Papillary serous variety
   C. Clear cell
   D. Adenosquamous

8. Which of the following type of Ca endometrium has the worst prognosis?
   A. Papillary serous variety
   B. Adenocarcinoma
   C. Clear cell
   D. Mucinous

9. Simpson's pain is seen in:
   A. Ca ovary
   B. Ca cervix
   C. Ca endometrium
   D. All of the above

10. All of the following are indications for postoperative radiotherapy in a case of carcinoma endometrium, except:
    A. Myometrial invasion > ½ thickness
    B. Positive lymph nodes
    C. Endocervical involvement
    D. Tumor positive for estrogen receptors

11. Choice of adjuvant treatment for endometrial carcinoma stage IA, grade I is:
    A. Radiotherapy
    B. Chemotherapy
    C. Chemotherapy plus radiotherapy
    D. Regular follow-up

12. Stage 2 Ca endometrium, treatment is:
    A. Radiotherapy
    B. Modified radical hysterectomy
    C. Modified radical hysterectomy followed by radiotherapy
    D. Chemotherapy

13. Endometrial Ca involving > 50% of myometrium, with vagina metastasis. No pelvic or para-aortic nodes involved. Peritoneal cytology is positive. Staging is:
    A. III a
    B. III b
    C. III c
    D. IV b

14. Carcinosarcoma can arise in:
    A. Uterus
    B. Fallopian tube
    C. Ovary
    D. All of the above

15. In grade 1 Ca endometrium, there is presence of ___% nonsqoumaous growth.
    A. ~5
    B. 6–25
    C. 25–50
    D. 50

16. Complex hyperplasia with atypia, will become cancerous in:
    A. 5%
    B. 10%
    C. 30%
    D. 50%

17. 30-year-old nulliparous has simple hyperplasia. The best treatment for her is:
    A. Simple hysterectomy
    B. Progesterone
    C. Estrogen
    D. Radical hysterectomy

18. 45-year-old P3L3 with complex hyperplasia with atypia, the best treatment is:
    A. Simple hysterectomy
    B. Progesterone
    C. Estrogen
    D. Radical hysterectomy

19. In a patient with postmenopausal bleeding, ET, more than ____ mm requires further evaluation.
    A. 1
    B. 2
    C. 3
    D. 4

20. Ca endometrium with inguinal lymph node involvement is stage __.
    A. II
    B. III
    C. IVb
    D. IV a

21. First line chemotherapy for endometrial cancer is:
    A. Rapamycin
    B. Doxorubicin
    C. Ifosfomide + Mesna
    D. Temsirolimus

22. In a woman 56 years old with first episode of post menopausal bleeding, following TVS findings are associated with endometrial cancer except:
    A. Thick endometrium > 9 mm
    B. In homogenous endometrium

C. Presence of fluid in the endometrial cavity

D. Endometrial thickness < 4 mm

23. Which of the following is true for MRI in postmenopausal bleeding?

A. It has high degree of sensitivity for endometrial carcinoma

B. It cannot predict myometrial invasion

C. It is a cheaper option than USG

D. It has high degree of specificity for endometrial carcinoma

Answer Key

1. C	5. A	9. C	13. B	17. B
2. A	6. C	10. D	14. D	18. A
3. D	7. A	11. D	15. A	19. D
4. B	8. C	12. C	16. C	20. C
				21. B
				22. D
				23. A

Explanations

1. **C** Rick factors for endometrial Ca:
   - Nulliparity
   - Early menarche, late menopause
   - Obesity
   - Diabetes mellitus and hypertension
   - PCOD
   - Unopposed estrogen therapy
   - Tamoxifen therapy
   - Atypical endometrial hyperplasia

2. **A** Type of hyperplasia progression to Ca (%)
   - Simple   1
   - Complex   3
   - Simple with atypia   8
   - Complex with atypia   29

3. **D** Obesity, hypertension, and diabetes mellitus associated with Ca endometrium = corpus cancer syndrome

4. **B** (Ovary) Different tissues tolerate different doses of radiation, but the ovaries are by far the most radiosensitive. They tolerate up to 2500 rad, while the other tissues listed tolerate between 5000 and 20,000 rad.

5. **A** Causes of postmenopausal uterine bleeding:
   Cause of bleeding percentage
   - Endometrial atrophy   60–80
   - Hormone replacement therapy   15–25
   - Endometrial polyps   2–12
   - Endometrial hyperplasia   5–10
   - Endometrial carcinoma   10

6. **C** Endometrial cancer most often occurs in the sixth and seventh decade of life, at an average age of 60 years.
   - 75% of cases occur in women older than 50 years of age.

7. **A** Adenocarcinoma is the most common variety of Ca endometrium.

8. **C** • Papillary serous variety and clear cell variety have worst prognosis.
   - Among the two, clear cell variety has poorer prognosis.

9. **C** Simpson's pain = colicky pain in patients of Ca endometrium.

10. **D** Tumor positive for estrogen receptors

11. **D** (No treatment) Management of Ca endometrium:
   - *Stage 1*: Surgery (total abdominal hysterectomy with bilateral salpingo-oophorectomy with lymph node sampling), followed by radiotherapy.
   - Only patients with stage 1A, grades 1 and 2 do not require postoperative radiotherapy.

12. **C** *Stage 2*: Modified radical hysterectomy, bilateral salpingo-oophorectomy with lymph node dissection, followed by radiotherapy.

    Stages 3 and 4: Debulking surgery followed by radiotherapy.

14. **D** (All of the above) A malignant mixed Mullerian tumor, also known as malignant mixed mesodermal tumor, MMMT and carcinosarcoma, is a malignant neoplasm found in the uterus, the ovaries, the fallopian tubes, and other parts of the body that contains both carcinomatous (epithelial tissue) and sarcomatous (connective tissue) components.

    It is divided into two types: homologous (in which the sarcomatous component is made of tissues found in the uterus such as endometrial, fibrous and/or smooth muscle tissues) and a heterologous type (made up of tissues not found in the uterus, such as cartilage, skeletal muscle, and/or bone). MMMT accounts for between 2 and 5% of all tumors derived from the body of the uterus, and are found predominantly in postmenopausal women with an average age of 66 years. Risk factors are similar to those of adenocarcinomas and include obesity, exogenous estrogen therapies, and nulliparity. Less well understood but potential risk factors include tamoxifen therapy and pelvic irradiation.

    In gross appearance, MMMTs are fleshier than adenocarcinomas, may be bulky and polypoid, and sometimes protrude through the cervical os. On histology, the tumors consist of adenocarcinoma (endometrioid, serous, or clear cell) mixed with the malignant mesenchymal (sarcoma) elements; alternatively, the tumor may contain two distinct and separate epithelial and mesenchymal components. Sarcomatous components may also mimic extrauterine tissues (e.g. striated muscle, cartilage, adipose tissue, and bone). Metastases usually contain only epithelial components.

Colonic Cancer

◙ *Seema Sharma*

1. In the women's health initiative estrogen plus progestin trial, estro-gen plus progestin use for an average of 5.6 years increased the risk of colorectal cancer among post- menopausal women with intact uterus.
   A. True
   B. False

2. In the estrogen alone arm of WHI these was no significant difference in the rates of colorectal cancer for conju-gated equine estrogen versus placebo.
   A. True
   B. False

3. Breast cancer detection demonstration project follow-up study by Troisi et al in 1997 suggested an inverse associa-tion between use of any menopausal hormone therapy and colorectal cancer risk.
   A. True
   B. False

4. According to recent research decrea-sing levels of ER-β coincide with the loss of differentiation of malignant colon cells thereby causing a protec-tive mechanism.
   A. True
   B. False

5. Age related CPG island methylation of the ER gene is not found in colorectal cancer.
   A. True
   B. False

6. All are true about colorectal cancer except:
   A. Largely preventable
   B. People who have a colonoscopy are 53% less likely to die from colon cancer over the next 15+ year
   C. Over 90% of people diagnosed with colon cancer are under 50 years
   D. Use of unopposed estrogen is associated with 15–46% reduction in risk of colon or colorectal cancer

7. Screening guidelines for colonoscopy include:
   A. Beginning at age 50 to be repeated every 10 years if the result are normal
   B. African American should start screening at 45 years
   C. Women 50 years and above should have yearly fecal occult blood test
   D. All of the above

8. HNPCC syndrome (hereditary non-polyposis colonic cancer) accounts for ---- of all colorectal cancer.
A. 2–5%
B. 85–90%
C. 15–20%
D. None of the above

9. HNPCC syndrome has following types:
A. Lynch I
B. Lynch II
C. Both A and B
D. None of the above

10. Following is true about HNPCC syndrome except:
A. It is inherited as an autosomal dominant syndrome

B. Over 90% of all colorectal cancers in HNPCC patients demostrate at least 2 or more mutated genes in HNPCC families or atypical HNPCC families

C. HNPCC presents at an older age than in the general population

D. It is characterized by an increased risk of other cancers, such as endometrial cancer, and gastrointestinal cancer

11. Mutations that are associated with Lynch syndrome (Hereditary Non Polyposis Colonic Cancer) are:
A. MSH2, MLH1, PMS1 and PMS2
B. MSH2, MLH1, PMS1, BRAC1
C. BRCA1, BRCA2, MSH2, PMS1
D. MLH1, PMS1, PMS2, BRCA2

Answer Key

1. B	3. A	5. B	7. D	9. C	11. A
2. A	4. A	6. C	8. A	10. C	

Explanation

HNPCC syndrome

"Hereditary nonpolyposis colorectal cancer (HNPCC) is the most common form of hereditary colorectal cancer. It is inherited as an autosomal dominant syndrome as a result of defective mismatch repair (MMR) proteins. HNPCC, accounts for 2–5% of all colorectal carcinomas. Over 90% of all colorectal cancers in HNPCC patients demonstrate a high microsatellite instability (MSI-H), which means at least 2 or more genes have been mutated in HNPCC families or atypical HNPCC families.

Colorectal cancer in patients with HNPCC presents at an earlier age than in the general population and is characterized by an increased risk of other cancers, such as endometrial cancer and, to a lesser extent, cancers of the ovary, stomach, small intestine, hepatobiliary tract, pancreas, upper urinary tract, prostrate, brain, and skin.

HNPCC is divided into Lynch syndrome I (familial colon cancer) and Lynch syndrome II (HNPCC associated with other cancers of the gastrointestinal [GI] or reproductive system). The increased cancer risk is due to inherited mutations that degrade the self-repair capability of DNA.

The tumor testing (i.e. immunohistochemistry, MSI, germline testing, and BRAF mutation testing), screening, and prophylactic surgery all help to reduce the risk of death in patients with HNPCC or Lynch syndrome.

The benefits of all strategies primarily affect relatives with a mutation associated with HNPCC or Lynch syndrome.

Screening for colorectal tumor testing helps to identify families with HNPCC or Lynch syndrome."
Reference: https://emedicine.medscape.com/article/188613-overview

Ovarian Carcinoma

◼ *Seema Sharma*

1. 54-year-old postmenopausal woman presents with bleeding per vaginum on ultrasound cystic solid mass 8 cm seen: most likely cause is:
   A. Hilus cell tumor
   B. Arrhenoblastoma
   C. Granulosa cell tumor
   D. Cystadenoma

2. Which of the following tumor markers is most likely to be raised in ovarian dysgerminoma?
   A. Serum HCG
   B. Serum α fetoprotein
   C. Serum lactic dehydrogenase
   D. Serum Inhibin

3. All of the following are known risk factors for the development of ovarian carcinoma except:
   A. Family H/O ovarian carcinoma
   B. Use of oral contraceptive pills
   C. Infertility treatment with clomiphene
   D. BRCA – 1 positive individual

4. Which of the following has a normal level of α fetoprotein value in serum?
   A. Ovarian dysgerminoma
   B. Hepatoblastoma
   C. Embryonal carcinoma
   D. Yolk sac tumor

5. About _____ % of ovarian neoplasms in postmenopausal women are malignant.
   A. 30
   B. 40
   C. 50
   D. 70

6. Which of these cancer does not have a National Health Service (NHS) screening programme?
   A. Ovarian cancer
   B. Breast cancer
   C. Bowel cancer
   D. Cervical cancer

7. Performance of prophylactic salpingo-oopherectomy reduces the risk of BRCA related gynaecologic cancer by:
   A. 50%
   B. 75%
   C. 90%
   D. 80%

8. Parity is inversely related to the risk of ovarian Ca, having at least one child is protective for disease, with the risk reduction of:
   A. 0.1 – 0.2
   B. 0.2 – 0.3
   C. 0.3 – 0.4
   D. 0.4 – 0.5

9. Which of the following indicates the chances of an ovarian cyst harboring malignancy?
  A. Morphologic indexing by ultrasound
  B. Ca 125
  C. RMI

D. All of the above

10. Which of the following values of RMI carry very high-risk for malignancy?
  A. > 25
  B. > 50
  C. > 250
  D. None of the above

Answer Key

1. C	3. B	5. A	7. D	9. D
2. C	4. A	6. A	8. C	10. C

Explanations and References

1. Jacobs I, Oram D, Fairbanks J, et al. A risk of malignancy index incorporating Ca 125, ultrasound and menopausal status for the accurate preoperative diagnosis of ovarian cancer. *Br J Obstet Gynaecol*. 1990; 97 (10): 922–9. Pubmed citation
2. Meys EM, Kaijser J, Kruitwagen RF, et al. Subjective assessment versus ultrasound models to diagnose ovarian cancer: A systematic review and meta-analysis. *Eur. J. Cancer*. 2016; 58: 17–29. doi:10.1016/j.ejca.2016.01.007 - Pubmed citation
9. **D** Morphologic indexing of a cyst is helpful to know if the cyst is malignant. Morphologic index developed by De priest is given below.[6]

Ultrasound score	1	2	3	4
Tumour volume	< 10 cm	10–50 cm	50–200 cm	> 200 cm
Cyst wall structure and wall thickness	Smooth < 3 mm	Smooth > 3 mm	Papillary < 3 mm	Papillary > 3 mm
Septal structure	No septa	Thin septa < 3 mm	Thick septa 3–10 mm	Solid area > 10 mm

A point scale (0 to 4) was developed within each category, with the total points per evaluation varying from 0 to 12.

An ultrasound morphology index score < 5 in a premenopausal woman is in keeping with a benign aetiology.

In postmenopausal patients, a morphology index score ≥ 5 has a positive predictive value for malignancy of 0.45.

10. **C** Risk of Malignancy Index (RMI) = U × M × Ca 125.

U = Ultrasound score

M = 3, a constant for menopausal women. (M is 1 for premenopausal women)

CA 125 = value of Ca 125.
  • Low-risk RMI = < 25; Risk of cancer is <3%
  • Moderate-risk RMI = 25 to 250; Risk of cancer is 20%;
  • High-risk RMI = > 250 Risk of cancer is 75%.

Sarcopenia

◾ *Suvarna Khadilkar*

1. Sarcopenia is defined as:
   A. Back pain with neurologic symptoms
   B. The loss of muscle mass and function associated with underlying disease
   C. The loss of muscle mass and function associated with aging
   D. None of the above

2. Consensus definition of sarcopenia by Europian working group on sarcopenia in older people (EWGSOP) of appendicular skeletal muscle mass index (ASMI) is:
   A. Below 6.2 kg/m²
   B. < 5.5 kg/m²
   C. Below 7.2 kg/m²
   D. None of the above

3. EWGSOP suggests a conceptual staging as:
   A. 'Presarcopenia', 'sarcopenia' and 'severe sarcopenia.'
   B. Mild, moderate, severe
   C. Stage I, stage II stage III
   D. Any of the above

4. Which of the following does not lead to sarcopenia?
   A. Decreased protein and energy intake
   B. Hypervitaminosis D
   C. Hypo-oestrogenism
   D. Genetic influence
   E. Immobility

5. Muscle mass proteins synthesis is dependent on all except:
   A. Exercise
   B. Testosterone
   C. IGF1, insulin
   D. PI3k /AKT- mTOR
   E. Myostatin

6. At menopause the musculoskeletal health is adversely affected because:
   A. Skeletal muscles have estrogen receptors
   B. Bones have estrogen receptors
   C. Oestrogen deficiency accelerates age related deterioration
   D. All of the above

7. According to EWGSOP, screening for sarcopenia is recommended in following:
   State true or false:
   A. Bedbound/ after hospitalization
   B. Shooting pain from back to leg
   C. Unable to rise from a sitting position unassisted
   D. History of weight loss (> 5%)
   E. Gymnasts

F. History of recurrent falls

G. Gait speed < 0.8 m/s over 4 m

8. Diagnosis of -----------is made when any 3 of the following 5 criteria are present in an individual.
   1. Unintentional weight loss
   2. Physical exhaustion
   3. Weakness (poor grip strength)
   4. Slow motor performance (walking speed)
   5. Low physical activity

   Choose correct diagnosis:
   A. Sarcopenia
   B. Sarcopenic obesity
   C. Frailty
   D. Sarco-osteoporosis

9. Diabetes and loss of muscle mass share following common etiological pathways except:
   A. Reduced physical activity
   B. Lower activity of anabolic hormones like insulin like growth factor–1, testosterone, Ghrelin
   C. The negative effects of diabetes on blood flow to muscle cells
   D. Increased energy intake

10. High incidence of morbidity and mortality is observed in:
    A. Osteosarcopenic obesity
    B. Sarcopenia
    C. Osteoporosis
    D. Osteoarthritis

11. Treatment of sarcopenia involves all except:
    A. Progressive resistance training (PRT)
    B. Calcium and vitamin D supplementation
    C. Decrease in protein and energy intake
    D. Minerals
    E. Lifestyle modification

12. Which of the following reduces the risk of falls?
    A. Vitamin D supplementation
    B. Walking stick
    C. Eyesight check-ups
    D. Hip joint support
    E. All of the above

13. Physically inactive adults after 30 can loose their muscle mass:
    A. 3–5%/year
    B. 3–5%/decade
    C. 10%/decade
    D. None of the above

14. Which statement is true about Sarcopenia at menopause?
    A. Judicious use of menopause hormone therapy (MHT) in early menopause may prevent sarcopenia in late menopause
    B. MHT has no effect on sarcopenia
    C. Sarcopenia is a feature of early menopause
    D. All of the above

Answer Key

1. C	5. E	C. True	G. True	11. C
2. B	6. D	D. True	8. C	12. E
3. A	7. A. **True**	E. False	9. D	13. B
4. B	B. False	F. True	10. A	14. A

References

1. Mithal A, et al. Osteoporosis International. 2013; 24(5):1555–66.
2. Keller K, et al. Muscles Ligaments Tendons Journal. 2014; 3(4):346–50.
3. Cruz-Jentoft AJ, et al. Age and Ageing. 2010; 39(4):412–23. Fried LP, Ferrucci L, Darrer J, Williamson JD, Anderson G. Untangling the concepts of disability, frailty and comorbidity: Implications for improved targeting and care. *J Gerontol A Biol Sci Med Sci*. 2004; 59(3):255–63.
5. Landi F, et al. Journal of the American Medical Directors Association.
6. Khandelwal D, et al. The Journal of Nutrition Health and Aging. 2012; 16(8):732–5.

Chapter

34

Osteoporosis

◉ *Rashmi Shah and Sudha Sharma*

1. How much approximately is skeletal calcium loss when it is picked up by conventional radiography?
   - **A.** 30–40%
   - **B.** 20–30%
   - **C.** 40–50%
   - **D.** 50–60%

2. Osteoporosis can cause bones to easily break and usually has no physical signs or symptoms. However, there is one clear sign which suggests that you should be tested for osteoporosis:
   - **A.** You feel pain in your legs and arms
   - **B.** You feel weak and tired
   - **C.** Your joints are stiff
   - **D.** You have lost more than 3 cm (just over an inch) in height

3. All of the following are risk factors for osteoporosis except:
   - **A.** Alcohol use
   - **B.** Smoking
   - **C.** Low calcium intake
   - **D.** Obesity
   - **E.** Turner's syndrome

4. Which of these factors raises osteoporosis risk in women?
   - **A.** Early menopause (before age 45)
   - **B.** Late menopause (after age 52)

   - **C.** Taking hormone replacement therapy
   - **D.** Having a BMI over 19 kg/m^2

5. Which of these diseases is associated with a greater risk of osteoporosis?
   - **A.** Rheumatoid arthritis
   - **B.** Gastrointestinal disorders such as Crohn's disease
   - **C.** Diabetes
   - **D.** All of the above

6. WHO criteria of – 2.5 SD below peak bone mass only apply for:
   - **A.** Non-DEXA techniques
   - **B.** DEXA techniques
   - **C.** Conventional radiography
   - **D.** Ultrasonography

7. Importance of measuring BMD:
   - **A.** Screening the high-risk population
   - **B.** Preventing the fractures
   - **C.** Diagnosing the fractures
   - **D.** None of the above

8. As per National Osteoporosis Foundation, when should we ask for BMD:
   - **A.** Women aged 65 and older
   - **B.** Men aged 65 and older
   - **C.** Postmenopausal women under age 70 with risk factor for fracture
   - **D.** Adults without a fragility fracture

9. In what conditions BMD measurement may not reflect accurate BMD:
   A. Laminectomy, calcification abdominal aorta
   B. Measuring BMD at spine, femoral neck
   C. Measuring BMD at hip
   D. Measuring BMD at forearm

10. In osteoporotic patients, BMD should be done after what interval to monitor change?
    A. 18–24 months
    B. 12–18 months
    C. 24–36 months
    D. 6–12 months

11. With each SD reduction in bone mass, there is a:
    A. Two fold increase in risk of fracture
    B. Three fold increase in risk of fracture
    C. Four fold increase in risk of fracture
    D. None of the above

12. In which of the following conditions can FRAX tool be used?
    A. Can be used without BMD when DEXA is not available
    B. Can be used in premenopausal patients
    C. Can be used to evaluate patients who are on treatment for osteoporosis
    D. All of the above

13. FRAX tool has limitations as it does not include certain risk factors such as:
    A. History of previous fractures
    B. Risk of falls
    C. History of glucocorticoid intake
    D. All of the above

14. FRAX predicts absolute risk for a fracture in an individual for:
    A. 10 years
    B. 8 years
    C. 4 years
    D. 6 years

15. Garvan risk calculator tool takes into consideration the following conditions except:
    A. History of prior fractures
    B. History of falls
    C. History of current alcohol intake and smoking
    D. BMD

16. All the following are bone resorption markers except:
    A. Hydroxyproline
    B. Pyridinoline and deoxypyridinoline
    C. Bone specific alkaline phosphatase
    D. N telopeptide-crosslinks of type I collagen

17. For bone resorption biochemical markers, best collection time is:
    A. Morning
    B. Afternoon
    C. Evening
    D. Night

18. All are metabolic or endocrine causes of osteoporosis except:
    A. Diabetes mellitus – Type II
    B. Hyperparathyroidism (primary)
    C. Hyperthyroidism
    D. Hypogonadism (primary and secondary)

19. Which is the WHO recommended diagnostic method for patients at risk of osteoporosis:
    A. Photometry
    B. Densitometry
    C. X-ray metry
    D. All of the above

20. As per WHO criteria T score of 1.5 will be diagnostic of:
    A. Osteoporosis
    B. Normal bone density
    C. Osteopenia
    D. None of the above

21. 25% mortality is associated with:
    A. Forearm fracture
    B. Vertebral fracture

C. Femur fracture

D. Rib fracture

22. Which of the following is a second generation bisphosphonate?
    A. Etidronate
    B. Alendronate
    C. Zolendronate
    D. None of the above

23. Which of the following does not cause osteoporosis?
    A. Crohn's disease
    B. Cushing's syndrome
    C. Obesity
    D. Stein-Leventhal syndrome

24. All of the following correctly describe denosumab except:

A. Reduces the incidence of vertebral fractures by about 68%

B. Approved for treatment of post-menopausal osteoporosis in women at high-risk of fracture

C. Increases the risk of cellulitis and skin rashes

D. Can cause hypercalcaemia

25. All of the following are primary goals of osteoporosis therapy according to NAMS position statement except:
    A. Prevent fractures
    B. Slowing or stopping bone loss
    C. Maintain bone strength
    D. Eliminate factors that may contribute to fractures
    E. Induce new bone synthesis

Answer Key

1. A	6. B	11. A	16. C	21. C
2. D	7. A	12. A	17. A	22. B
3. D	8. A	13. B	18. A	23. D
4. A	9. A	14. A	19. B	24. D
5. D	10. B	15. C	20. C	25. E

Reference

8. Cosman AF, de Beur SJ, LeBoff MS, Lewiecki EM, Tanner B, Randall S, Lindsay R (2014). Clinician's Guide to Prevention and Treatment of Osteoporosis. Osteoporosis International, 25(10), 2359–81. http:// doi.org/10.1007/s00198-014-2794-2

Treatment of Osteoporosis

◙ *Sudha Sharma*

1. Bisphosphonates have a half-life of:
   A. > 10 years
   B. < 10 years
   C. = 10 years
   D. None

2. Bisphosphonates act to:
   A. Inhibit bone resorption
   B. Stimulate bone formation
   C. Both
   D. None

3. Alendronate reduces the risk of vertebral fractures by approximately
   A. 40%
   B. 50%
   C. 60%
   D. 70%

4. Alendronate reduces the risk of hip and wrist fracture by approximately
   A. 10%
   B. 20%
   C. 30%
   D. 40%

5. Risedronate when discontinued, the beneficial effect on BMD and markers of bone tumour appear to revert partially or completely within:
   A. 1 years
   B. 2 years

   C. 3 years
   D. 4 years

6. Ibandronate is approved for the prevention and treatment of postmenopausal osteoporosis:
   A. True
   B. False

7. A once monthly formulation of ibandronate is available in dosage of:
   A. 100 mg
   B. 200 mg
   C. 150 mg
   D. 50 mg

8. Zolendronic acid (5 mg) to be administered:
   A. Half yearly
   B. Yearly
   C. 2 yearly
   D. None

9. Zolendronic acid (5 mg) must be infused over:
   A. 5 minutes
   B. 10 minutes
   C. 15 minutes
   D. 20 minutes

10. All bisphosphonates are not recommended if GFR is:
    A. < 35 ml/minute

B. < 45 ml/minute

C. < 55 ml/minute

D. None

11. Bisphosphonates have been associated with which side effect?
    A. GI reflux, musculoskeletal pain
    B. Osteonecrosis jaw
    C. Atypical fracture femur
    D. Ocular pain
    E. All of the above

12. Teriparatide treatment is recommended for treatment of:
    A. Osteopenia
    B. Osteoporosis
    C. Severe osteoporosis
    D. None of the above

13. Following two statements are true or false:
    1. Sustained elevation of parathyroid hormone leads to bone resorption.
    2. Intermittent administration of PTH stimulates bone formation more than resorption.
    A. True
    B. False

14. Bone formation begins within ------ months of administration of PTH.
    A. 4
    B. 3
    C. 2
    D. 1

15. The action of PTH on skeletal compartments are:
    A. Receptor specific
    B. Site specific
    C. Both A and B
    D. None of the above

16. Dosage of PTH is:
    A. 10 mcg/day SC
    B. 20 mcg/day SC
    C. 30 mcg/day IM
    D. 40 mcg/day IV

17. PTH is not recommended for use beyond:
    A. 4 years

B. 3 years

C. 2 years

D. 1 year

18. All are side effects of PTH except:
    A. Hypotension, nausea
    B. Myalgia, arthralgia
    C. Hypercalcemia, hyperuricemia
    D. Hypertension, uraemia

19. Strontium ranelate has been shown to have properties as:
    A. Anabolic and antiresorptive
    B. Anabolic
    C. Antiresorptive
    D. None of the above

20. Strontium ranelate has been shown to reduce:
    A. Vertebral fractures
    B. Nonvertebral fractures
    C. Both
    D. None

21. Following are the side effects of strontium ranelate except:
    A. Diarrhoea
    B. Venous and pulmonary thromboembolism
    C. Severe skin reactions
    D. Headache and hypotension

22. Raloxifene is used for:
    A. Prevention of osteoporosis
    B. Treatment of osteoporosis
    C. Both prevention and treatment
    D. None

23. Raloxifene is recommended in the dosage of:
    A. 60 mg/day
    B. 70 mg/day
    C. 50 mg/day
    D. 40 mg/day

24. Raloxifene is beneficial for simultaneous reduction of invasive breast cancer by:
    A. 50%
    B. 76%
    C. 40%
    D. 60%

25. Raloxifene should be used in perimenopausal and early post-menopausal females:

A. True
B. False

Answer Key

1. A	6. A	11. E	16. B	21. D
2. A	7. C	12. C	17. C	22. C
3. C	8. B	13. A	18. A	23. A
4. A	9. C	14. C	19. A	24. C
5. A	10. A	15. C	20. C	25. B

References

1-25   Rosen HN, Drezner MK, Rosen CJ, Schmader KE, Mulder JE. Overview of the management of osteoporosis in postmenopausal women. Monografía en Internet. Up to date. 2017.

4   **A.** Papapoulos SE, Quandt SA, Liberman UA, Hochberg MC, Thompson DE. Meta-analysis of the efficacy of alendronate for the prevention of hip fractures in postmenopausal women. Osteoporos Int. 2005 May; 16(5):468–74.

Iwamoto J, Sato Y, Takeda T, Matsumoto H. Hip fracture protection by alendronate treatment in postmenopausal women with osteoporosis: a review of the literature. Clinical interventions in aging. 2008 Sep;3(3):483.

Osteoarthritis

◾ *Seema Sharma*

1. Osteoarthritis is characteristically rapidly progressing disease affecting multiple joints in a few days duration.
   A. True
   B. False

2. Levels of acute phase reactants in patients with osteoarthritis are found:
   A. Very high
   B. In reference range
   C. Very low
   D. Mildly raised

3. The plain radiography is the imaging method of choice for osteoarthritis-
   A. True
   B. False

4. On plain radiography features of primary osteoarthritis are:
   A. Abnormalities found in load bearing areas
   B. Loss of joint spaces
   C. Subchondral bony sclerosis and cyst formation
   D. All of the above
   E. None of the above

5. Which of the following is not true for bone scanning in osteoarthritis:
   A. Can be helpful in early diagnosis of osteoarthritis of hand

   B. Yield a symmetrically patterned very mildly increased uptake
   C. Can differentiate multiple myeloma from osteoarthritis
   D. Cannot be of help in differentiating osteoarthritis from osteomyelitis and bone metastases

Case Scenarios: Osteoarthritis

CASE 1: A 55 years old postmenopausal female presented with deep, achy pain in right knee which is exacerbated by extensive use. On examination the range of movement is reduced, and crepitus are frequently present. She also complains of morning joint stiffness lasting for less than 30 seconds.

6. Most appropriate clinical diagnosis for her is:
   A. Gouty arthritis
   B. Lyme disease
   C. Osteoarthritis
   D. Avascular necrosis

7. Diagnosis for her can be made on the basis of clinical and radiographic evidence.
   A. True
   B. False

8. All of the following are considered as osteoarthritic indicators by researches except:
   A. Monoclonal antibodies
   B. Synovial fluid markers
   C. Urinary pyridinium cross links
   D. C-reactive protein

9. The Synovial fluid analysis for her is expected to show:
   A. WBC < 2000/µL with mononuclear predominance
   B. WBC < 2000/µL with eosinophilic predominance
   C. WBC > 10,000 with mononuclear predominance
   D. WBC > 20,000

10. Which of the following is not advisable as non-pharmacological interventions for her?
    A. Cold therapy
    B. Weight loss

C. Unloading of joint
D. Avoidance of exercise

CASE 2: A 54 years old female presents with pain and difficulty in movement of left elbow joint.

11. Which of the following is true?
    A. Elbow joint is a common site of osteoarthritis
    B. CT scanning is the most useful modality for guiding her diagnosis
    C. Elbow arthritis can occur because of previous trauma in her elbow
    D. Joint replacement is the 1st line therapy for this patient

12. Which of the following can best differentiate her osteoarthritis from inflammatory arthritis?
    A. SC reactive protein
    B. CT scan
    C. Arthrocentesis
    D. Bone scan

Answer Key

| 1. B | 3. A | 5. D | 7. A | 9. A | 11. C |
| 2. B | 4. D | 6. C | 8. D | 10. D | 12. C |

Case Scenarios: Osteoporosis

◼ *Seema Sharma*

CASE 1: A 68-year-old woman presented to accident and emergency department with right wrist pain, swelling and displacement following a trivial fall on outstretched hand during gardening on examination there was no open wound. She gives history of smoking.

1. Most likely diagnosis for her is:
   A. Intra-articular fracture of ulna
   B. Scaphoid fracture
   C. Colle's fracture
   D. Displacement of wrist joint

2. The most likely cause of this fracture:
   A. Primary osteoporosis
   B. Secondary osteoporosis
   C. Idiopathic
   D. Undiagnosed malignancy

3. The most common sites for osteoporotic fractures in postmenopausal women are:
   A. Vertebral, wrist and hips
   B. Vertebral, ankle and hips
   C. Ankle, wrist and hips
   D. Ankle, hips and wrist

4. Which of the following is true regarding life time risk of osteoporotic fractures?
   A. Spine – 30%
   B. Wrist – 15%

C. Hip – 40%
D. None of the above

5. Which of the following is not correct for her management?
   A. Start recommended dose of calcium and vitamin D_3
   B. Start lifestyle modification, e.g. diet and exercise
   C. Counsel her that a wrist facture is not a serious issue just be careful not to fall in future
   D. Stop smoking

CASE 2: A 72 years old menopausal woman presented to you with loss of balance and buckling since 2 years. Difficulty in maintaining same posture for more than 15–20 minutes and general body fatigue.

6. What is the most recommended bone mineral density test for her?
   A. DEXA (dual energy X-ray absorptiometry) to measure BMD at the spine and hip
   B. BMD (bone mineral density)
   C. QUS (quantitative ultrasound to measure BMD at the heel or finger)
   D. A simple blood test to measure calcium in blood

7. Her T score on dexa was '–4' what would be the first option of therapy?
   A. Alendronate
   B. Only calcium and vitamin D
   C. Teriparatide
   D. Strontium

8. If lifestyle modifications and exercises were advised, which of the following exercise is not of specific benefit for bone health?
   A. Using weights or doing other resistance and muscle strengthening exercises
   B. Swimming
   C. Jogging, walking
   D. Dancing

9. How will you monitor the response to the therapy after two years?
   A. Bone resorption markers
   B. Repeat DEXA
   C. Both A and B
   D. No need to monitor

10. Which of the following diseases is associated with a greater risk of osteoporosis?
    A. Diabetes
    B. Rheumatoid arthritis
    C. Crohn's disease
    D. All of the above

11. **CASE 3:** A 70-year-old woman presented with severe body pain. Her bone mineral density was low. She had a past history of a transient ischemic attack best therapy for her would be:
    A. Alendronate
    B. Calcium and vitamin D
    C. Isoflavones
    D. None of the above

12. **CASE 4:** A 55-year-old woman presented with hot flushes. She had vaginal dryness and weak bones. She had just recovered from an osteoporotic bone fracture. Drug of choice for her is:
    A. Raloxifene
    B. Bazidoxifene and conjugated estrogen
    C. Calcium and vitamin D
    D. Both B and C

13. **CASE 5:** A 62-year-old lady presented with body pain and recurrent osteoporotic fractures. Her T score was –4.5 she had been treated for breast cancer. Best plan for her treatment would be:
    A. Menopausal hormone therapy
    B. Injection teriparatide for a year followed by raloxifene treatment
    C. Only calcium and vitamin D
    D. None of the above

14. **CASE 6:** A 40-year-old perimenopausal woman presented with severe hot flushes. She was not willing for hormonal treatment because she had a family histroy of breast cancer. Treatment of choice for her is:
    A. Isoflavons
    B. Raloxifene
    C. Tamoxifene
    D. None of the above

Answer Key

1. C	4. B	7. C	10. D	13. B
2. A	5. C	8. B	11. B	14. A
3. A	6. A	9. B	12. D	

Explanations

7. **C** Teriparatide: This is the only bone stimulating drug others are antiresorptive so for a severe case like this a course of teriparatide 20 mcg subcutaneously for period of maximum 2 years is ideal thereafter to be followed up with bisphosphonates.

8. **B** Swimming is not a weight bearing exercise so its not so beneficial for osteoporosis.

9. **B** DEXA should be done after two years for assessing the therapy response in such severe cases of osteoporosis BMD should generally show improvement by at least 1–2 points and resorption markers also should show improved levels but markers should be done every 3–4 months and if no improvement molecule should be changed after reinvestigating any missing diagnosis of secondary osteoporosis.

12. **D** Raloxifene should not be used as patient has hot flushes.

13. **B** For severe case like this a course of teriparatide 20 mcg subcutaneously for period of maximum 2 years is ideal thereafter to be followed up with bisphosphonates, but since she has a h/o breast cancer, raloxifene is better option than bisphosphonates.

14. **A** Raloxifene and tamoxifene are not to be used as patient has hot flushes. Ideal would have been hormonal therapy but since patient is scared even after counselling, then isoflavons are the options with limited evidence.

Desmopressin and Diosmin

◉ *Jyoti Jaiswal*

1. Following is true for desmopressin except:
   - A. Desmopressin is a synthetic analogue of hormone vasopressin
   - B. It alters local hemostasis by increasing vascular uterine resistance
   - C. It exerts myometrial vasoconstrictor action
   - D. It can be used in treatment of IUD related menorrhagia

2. Desmopressin is contraindicated in patients with all except:
   - A. Renal failure
   - B. Hyponatremia
   - C. Hypertension
   - D. Decreased intracranial pressure

3. Citrus bioflavonoids and related substances are used to treat following disease except:
   - A. Acute venous insufficiency
   - B. Hemorrhoids
   - C. Nose bleed
   - D. Leg ulcers

4. Following statement is false:
   - A. Breast cancer surgery can lead to lymphoedema
   - B. Citrus bioflavonoids can decrease the swelling due to lymphoedema
   - C. Use of diosmin and hesperidin is done in 70:30 ratio
   - D. None of the above

5. While treating breast cancer the citrus bioflavonoid tangerine:
   - A. May reduce effectiveness of tamoxifen
   - B. May increase effectiveness of tamoxifen
   - C. No effect on effectiveness if tamoxifen
   - D. None of the above

Answer Key

| 1. B | 2. D | 3. A | 4. C | 5. A |

Ulipristal and Mifepristone

◙ *Priya Vora/Thakur*

1. Ulipristal causes all except:
   A. The increase in fibroid size
   B. The reduction in fibroid volume
   C. Decreases uterine bleeding
   D. Improves haemoglobin and haema-tocrit levels

2. Ulipristal acts by causing all except:
   A. Induces apoptosis
   B. Decreases angiogenesis
   C. Increases cell proliferation
   D. Suppressive action on endometrial vasculature

3. Ulipristal is a:
   A. SPRM
   B. SERM
   C. NSAID
   D. Progestin

4. Ulipristal is contraindicated in all except:
   A. Pregnancy
   B. Genital bleeding of undiagnosed etiology
   C. Uterine, cervical, breast cancer
   D. Perimenopausal women

5. Ulipristal should be started:
   A. Any day of menstrual cycle
   B. From day 1 to 7 of menstrual cycle only

   C. Any day during menses with or without food
   D. From day 3 to 5 of menstrual cycle only

6. Full form of PEARL is:
   A. PGL40001 efficacy assessment in reduction of symptoms due to uterine leiomyoma
   B. PGL4001 efficacy assessment in reduction of symptoms due to uterine leiomyoma
   C. PGL 401 efficacy assessment in reduction of symptoms due to uterine leiomyoma
   D. PGL 400001 efficacy assessment in reduction of symptoms due to uterine leiomyoma

7. Ulipristal acetate has a specific pharmacodynamic action on:
   A. Endometrium
   B. Cervix
   C. Fallopian tubes
   D. Ovaries

8. Ulipristal interacts with
   A. CYP3A4 inhibitors
   B. CYP3A4 inducers

C. Hormonal contraceptives and progestogens

D. All of the above

9. Ulipristal can cause undesirable effects like:
   A. Endometrial thickening
   B. Hot flushes
   C. Headache
   D. All of the above

10. Absorption of ulipristal occurs after:
    A. Approximately 2 hours after ingestion
    B. Approximately 1 hour after ingestion
    C. Approximately 24 hours after ingestion
    D. Approximately 1 hour after ingestion only when taken with food

11. Mifepristone has the following advantages over other therapies except:
    A. As effective as GnRh analogues
    B. No effect on BMD/risk of osteoporosis
    C. Oral route of administration with good compliance
    D. Greater side effects

12. All are true for mifepristone except:
    A. Should be taken within first seven days of menstrual cycle
    B. Should be taken at same time everyday
    C. Minimum duration 3–6 months
    D. On alternate days

13. Mifepristone caused all except:
    A. Increase in fibroid volume (26–74)%
    B. Amenorrhoea in 63–100%
    C. Reduces rates of menorrhagia and dysmenorrhea
    D. Some reports show reduction in the fibroid volume

14. Up to what fibroid size can mifepristone be prescribed?
    A. 3 to 12 cm
    B. 5–15 cm

C. 2.5–15 cm
D. 2.5–12 cm

15. When should mifepristone be started in relation to the menstrual cycle?
    A. 1st to 3rd day
    B. 7th to 14th day
    C. 1st to 7th day
    D. After ovulation

16. Mifepristone acts on fibroids by causing:
    A. Increase in apoptosis, decrease in angiogenesis, decrease in proliferation
    B. Decrease in apoptosis, increase in angiogenesis, increase in proliferation
    C. Increase in apoptosis, decrease in angiogenesis, increase in proliferation
    D. Decrease in apoptosis, decrease in angiogenesis, increase in proliferation

17. Medical treatment of fibroids includes all except:
    A. GnRh analogues
    B. Mifepristone
    C. Danazol
    D. Oral contraceptive pills

18. Mifepristone belongs to which class of drug:
    A. NSAID (non-steroidal anti-inflammatory drugs)
    B. SERM (selective estrogen receptors modulators)
    C. SPRM (selective progesterone receptor modulators)
    D. Progestins

19. Mifepristone interacts with:
    A. Corticosteroids
    B. Azole antifungals
    C. Erythromycin
    D. All of the above

20. All the characteristic histologic features are present in progesterone

receptor modulator associated endometrial changes except:

A. Cyst like dilatations in the endometrial glands

B. Abnormal vasculature

C. Changes in glandular connective tissue relationship

D. Malignant transformation of the endometrium

Answer Key

1. A	5. C	9. D	13. A	17. D
2. C	6. B	10. B	14. C	18. C
3. A	7. A	11. D	15. C	19. D
4. D	8. D	12. D	16. A	20. D

Non-Hormonal Treatment of Abnormal Uterine Bleeding (AUB)

▣ *Siddhesh Iyer and Suvarna Khadilkar*

1. What are the choices in non-hormonal medical therapies?
   A. Mefenamic acid
   B. Ethamsylate
   C. Tranexamic acid
   D. All of the above

2. All dosages of the following non-steroidal anti-inflammatory drugs (NSAIDs) are correct except?
   A. Mefenamic acid – 500 mg — TID
   B. Ibuprofen — 400 mg – TID
   C. Meclofenamate — 300 mg — TID
   D. Naproxen sodium — loading dose 550 mg then 275 mg 6 hourly

3. When do you start NSAIDs?
   A. Treatment is started with onset of bleeding and continued for 3–5 days as necessary
   B. Treatment is started two days before the onset of menses
   C. Once started, it is continued for 15 days irrespective of bleeding
   D. None of the above

4. How much percentage of reduction of blood loss can be expected with NSAIDs?
   A. 50–60%
   B. 25–30%

   C. 60–80 %
   D. None of the above

5. What are the contraindications for NSAIDs?
   A. Bleeding and platelet disorders
   B. Acute gastrointestinal disorders, such as ulcers
   C. Intolerance to NSAIDs or asthma
   D. All of the above

6. Which non-hormonal non-steroidal drug is used as a contraceptive as well as in AUB?
   A. Ormeloxifene
   B. Meclofenamate
   C. Raloxifene
   D. None of the above

7. What is the mechanism of action of ormeloxifene?
   A. It blocks the cytosol receptor by its competitive binding affinity over estradiol
   B. It not only causes a slow build-up of receptors but also causes their prolonged retention
   C. It has an antagonist action on estrogen receptors in uterus and breast
   D. All of the above

8. What is the dosage schedule of ormeloxifene for AUB treatment?

A. 60 mg tablet twice a week for first 12 weeks, then 60 mg/week for up to next 12 weeks

B. 30 mg twice a week for first 12 weeks followed by 30 mg/week

C. 120 mg twice a week for first 12 weeks, then 60 mg / week for next 12 weeks

D. None of the above

9. What is the dosage schedule of tranexamic acid as recommended in AUB?

A. 500 mg 6 hourly during the first four days of the cycle, or 25–50 mg/ kg daily by continuous infusion

B. 1000 mg 6 hourly during the first four days of the cycle, or 15 mg/kg daily by continuous infusion

C. 1000 mg 6 hourly during the first four days of the cycle, or 25–50 mg/ kg daily by continuous infusion

D. None of the above

10. What are the contraindications of tranexamic use?

A. Severe renal failure

B. Thromboembolic disease

C. Colour vision disorders

D. All of the above

11. What is not true about use of ethamsylate in AUB?

A. Ethamsylate (2,5-dihydroxy-benzene-sulfonate diethylammonium salt) is a synthetic hemostatic drug

B. It acts on the first step of hemostasis by improving platelet adhesiveness and restoring capillary resistance

C. It promotes P-selectin-dependent, platelet adhesive mechanisms

D. It is highly effective in menorrhagia treatment

12. Comparative success rates of various medical therapies in AUB are:

A. NSAIDs 25%

B. Tranexamic acid 50%

C. Progesterone therapy 80–90%

D. All are correct

13. A 45-year-old with heavy menstrual bleeding (HMB) and dysmenorrhoea since 3 months is being reviewed in clinic. Ultrasound shows no significant uterine abnormality. The patient has no significant past medical history and is not asthmatic. The patient not keen to use hormonal treatment. The best treatment for the patient is:

A. Levonorgestrel releasing system

B. Tranexamic acid

C. NSAIDs

D. Both B and C

14. A 42-year-old with heavy menstrual bleeding is being reviewed in clinic. She reports painful periods and states this is having a significant impact on her quality of life. Ultrasound shows 2 fibroids measuring 3.3 and 3.5 cm. The patient has no significant past medical history and is not asthmatic. She wants to avoid surgery. Which is the best option for her ?

A. Levonorgestrel-releasing intra-uterine system

B. Tranexamic acid

C. Uterine artery embolization

D. Endometrial ablation

Answer Key

1. D	4. B	7. D	10. D	13. D
2. C	5. D	8. A	11. D	14. C
3. A	6. A	9. C	12. D	

Hormonal Management AUB

☑ *Siddesh Iyer and Suvarna Khadilkar*

1. Which of the following statements is incorrect regarding levonorgestrel releasing intrauterine system:
   A. There is increased incidence of menorrhagia
   B. This system can be used as hormone replacement therapy
   C. This method is useful for the treatment of endometrial hyperplasia
   D. Irregular uterine bleeding can be a problem initially

2. A 42-year-old woman (parity 3) presents with menorrhagia. Considering she has no uterine pathology and is seeking an effective long-term reversible form of contraception, what would you suggest?
   A. Etonogestrel implant
   B. Gonadotrophin-releasing hormone agonists
   C. Injectable long-acting progestogens
   D. Levonorgestrel-releasing intrauterine device

3. Implanon contains:
   A. Ethinyl estradiol
   B. Etonogestrel
   C. Medroxy progesterone
   D. Gestodene

4. One of your junior colleagues wants to know about the pharmacological treatments for fibroid uterus. Which of the following is the appropriate explanation?
   A. LNG-IUS acts mainly by reduction of the fibroid size
   B. There is a specific histological appearance of the endometrium, which appears with the use of ulipristal acetate (UA) and persists for a year after stopping the treatment
   C. UA induces apoptosis in fibroid cells and inhibition of cellular proliferation
   D. When compared to GnRh analogues, UA controls menstrual blood loss less rapidly

5. LNG-IUS delivers:
   A. 20 mcg daily
   B. 30 mcg daily
   C. 50 mcg daily
   D. 55 mcg daily

6. Danazol is:
   A. Progesterone antagonist
   B. Androgenic steroid
   C. Estrogen precursor
   D. SERM

7. Ormeloxifen is:
   A. Selective estrogen receptor modulator (SERM)
   B. Selective progesterone receptor modulator (SPRM)
   C. Selective tissue estrogenic activity regulator (STEAR)
   D. Estrogen

8. LNG-IUS has to be changed every:
   A. 3 years
   B. 5 years
   C. 10 years
   D. 7 years

9. GnRh is associated with:
   A. Bone loss
   B. Heavy bleeding
   C. Migraine'
   D. Hirsutism

10. Side effect of depot medroxy progesterone is:
    A. Weight loss
    B. Irregular bleeding
    C. Hirsutism
    D. Endometrial hyperplasia

11. Following are the specific hormones used for managing AUB except:
    A. Oestrogen and progestins
    B. Levothyroxine
    C. GnRh agonists
    D. Androgens
    E. Tranexamic acid
    F. Desmopressin

12. Before starting hormonal treatment all of the following need to be ruled out except:

A. Polyps, adenomyosis, malignant premalignant changes
B. Bleeding disorders: von Willebrands disease
C. Contraindications for oestrogen and progestins treatment
D. History of thromboembolism
E. Pulmonary pathology
F. Uncontrolled hypertension, diabetes mellitus

13. Which of the following progestogens have the best hemostatic property in treatment of menorrhagia?
    A. Norethisterone
    B. Medroxyprogesterone
    C. Dydrogesterone
    D. Micronised progesterone

14. Estrogen only therapy is preferred in which of the following endometrial histopathologies in AUB?
    A. Endometrium proliferative phase
    B. Endometrium in cystic glandular hyperplasia
    C. Endometrium in simple hyperplasia
    D. Atrophic endometrium

15. In menorrhagia associated with hypothyroidism, option for definitive treatment is:
    A. Levothyroxine
    B. Mefenamic acid
    C. Thyroidectomy
    D. Tranexamic acid

Answers

1. A	4. C	7. A	10. B	13. A
2. D.	5. A	8. B	11. E	14. D
3. B	6. B	9. A	12. E	15. A

Recent Advances and Newer Techniques in AUB

■ *Deepali Prakash Kale and Siddhesh Iyer*

1. The favourable prognostic indicator for endometrial ablation is:
   A. Genuine heavy menstrual bleeding (HMB)
   B. Regular uterine cavity
   C. Cavity less than 12 cm
   D. H/O chronic pelvic pain

2. All are second generation techniques of endometrial ablation except:
   A. Transcervical resection of endo-metrium
   B. Thermal balloon endometrial ablation (TBEA)
   C. Impedance controlled bipolar radiofrequency endometrial ablation
   D. Endometrial laser intrauterine thermal therapy (ELITT)

3. Patients with following clinical profile can be offered endometrial ablation:
   A. 42 year P2L2 permanent sterilisa-tion done with heavy menstrual bleeding
   B. 37-year-old female with heavy menstrual bleeding with primary infertility
   C. 45-year-old female P1L1 with heavy menstrual bleeding not keen for further conception
   D. A and C

4. MRI has an advantage over USG in work-up of fibroids:
   A. Useful for identifying large fibroids
   B. Allows visualisation of ovaries in cases of large fibroids
   C. Adenomyosis
   D. All of the above

5. Following are complications of uterine arterial embolization:
   A. Pseudo-aneurysm of femoral artery
   B. Reactions to contrast media
   C. Both A and B
   D. None

6. True statement regarding MR focused USG is:
   A. Causes no significant decrease in menstrual blood loss
   B. Affects ovarian function
   C. Enables local treatment of fibroids with some shrinkage
   D. Discomfort is a major side effect

7. Mrs XY 48-year-old P3L3 is due to undergo a impedance controlled bipolar radiofrequency endome-trial ablation for heavy menstrual bleeding. Which is not true about this treatment?
   A. She need not be posted for hystero-scopic visualization

B. Endometrial pre-treatment with GnRh is a must before this procedure

C. Her histopathology report should be done before procedure

D. Time required for this procedure is 90 to 120 seconds, after which device is switched off automatically

8. Following types of submucous uterine fibroid as per palm coein classification are amenable for treatment by hysteroscopy except:
   A. Type 1
   B. Type 0
   C. Type 2
   D. Type 3

9. The artery which is usually cannulated in the procedure of uterine artery embolization?
   A. External iliac artery
   B. Internal iliac artery
   C. Femoral artery
   D. Obturator artery

10. The advantage of GnRh treatment prior to myomectomy are all except:
    A. Reduction in fibroid volume
    B. Increase in the preoperative haemoglobin levels
    C. Loss of plane between fibroid and the myometrium
    D. Useful in treatment of patients opting for conservative management of fibroids

11. A 41-year-old woman with three children presents with menorrhagia, without significant dysmenorrhoea, that has not responded to 6 months of Mirena therapy. Hysteroscopy showed a normal-shaped uterine cavity with cavity length of 10 cm. No intracavity fibroids or polyps were identified. She does not seek future fertility. What is the best treatment option, with the lowest risk?

A. Uterine artery embolisation
B. Total laparoscopic hysterectomy
C. Abdominal or vaginal hysterectomy
D. Endometrial ablation

12. LNG-IUS D contains following amount of levonorgestrel:
    A. 52 mg
    B. 20 mcg
    C. 40 mg
    D. 50 mcg

13. When used for treatment of AUB, LNG-IUS should be changed after?
    A. 2 years
    B. 3 years
    C. 4 years
    D. 5 years

14. Which of the following is an indication for endometrial ablation?
    A. Desire for fertility
    B. Women with a desire to preserve uterus
    C. Endometrial hyperplasia
    D. Postmenopausal women

15. Which of the following are contraindications for endometrial ablation?
    A. Endometrial hyperplasia
    B. Desire for fertility
    C. Large uterus (>12 cm cavity length)
    D. Suspected malignancy of the genital tract
    E. Multiple or large myomas
    F. All of the above

16. Which is true about the generations of the endometrial ablation techniques?
    A. Second generation techniques do not use heat as the ablative energy
    B. The first generation procedures do not need hysteroscopy guidance
    C. Second generation techniques can give tissue for histopathology
    D. Second generation techniques do not need hysteroscopy guidance

17. The following is a second generation ablation technique:
    A. Radiofrequency induced ablation
    B. Hydrothermablation
    C. Laser interstitial therapy
    D. All of the above

18. Dose of ormeloxifene for abnormal uterine bleeding is:
    A. 30 mg once weekly for 12 weeks
    B. 30 mg twice weekly for 6 weeks
    C. 60 mg once a week for 6 weeks
    D. 60 mg twice a week for 12 weeks

19. Complications of endometrial ablation:
    A. Uterine perforation
    B. Fluid overload
    C. Hemorrhage
    D. All the above

20. Temperature used in thermal balloon ablation technique is:
    A. 99°
    B. 87°
    C. 120°
    D. 100°

Answer Key

1. C	5. C	9. C	13. D	17. D
2. A	6. C	10. C	14. B	18. D
3. D	7. B	11. D	15. F	19. D
4. D	8. D	12. A	16. D	20. B

Explanations

7. **B** This procedure does not require pre treatment with GnRH or any such medication as Endometrium is a low impedance tissue is vaporized and removed by suction in the device. Suction improves the contact of the device with endometrium, increasing the effect of ablation. Radiofrequency energy desiccates and coagulates the endometrium and underlying superficial myometrium. Hence no tissue can be obtained for histopathology examination, hence prior histopathology should be done.

11. **D** The answer is endometrial ablation. Compared with hysterectomy, endometrial ablation is quicker to perform and results in shorter hospital stays and a faster return to work. Hysterectomy on the other hand, results in more adverse effects and is more expensive. It should be noted that the need for retreatment in endometrial ablation (approximately 20% over 5 years) leads its differential benefits to decrease over time.

Hysterectomy

☑ *Siddesh Iyer*

1. A 50-year-old woman had LNG IUS inserted 2 years ago for heavy menstrual periods. She was initially amenorrhoeic but has now developed heavy menstrual bleeding again. Endometrial biopsy shows endometrial hyperplasia with atypia. What is the best treatment option for her?
   A. Oral contraceptive pills in addition to LNG-IUS *in situ*
   B. Reinsert LNG-IUS
   C. Total abdominal hysterectomy and bilateral salpingo-oophorectomy
   D. Tranexamic acid in addition to LNG-IUS

2. A 47-year-old Para 3 who has had three previous vaginal deliveries presents with a history of HMB that has not responded to medical treatment or the levonorgestrel-containing intra-uterine system (LNG-IUS). The patient was offered endometrial ablation but declined. On examination, the uterus is bulky, no masses palpable in the adnexa and the cervix descends to about 2 cm above the hymenal ring. An ultrasound confirms the physical examination findings. What is the most appropriate treatment option?

   A. A combination of endometrial resection and levonorgestrel releasing-IUS
   B. Laparoscopic vaginal assisted hysterectomy as it enables the surgeon to assess the pelvic organs
   C. Total abdominal hysterectomy as there is a lower risk of bladder injury than a vaginal hysterectomy
   D. Vaginal hysterectomy

3. What treatment would you suggest for a 44-year-old woman with a completed family and 28-week size fibroid uterus who is complaining of menorrhagia, chronic abdominal pain, bowel and bladder obstructive symptoms?
   A. Abdominal hysterectomy
   B. Vaginal hysterectomy
   C. Uterine artery embolization
   D. OC PILLS

4. A 42-year-old woman is seeking a hysterectomy for persistent menorrhagia that has been unresponsive to endometrial ablation. She is parity 3, has a normal sized uterus and second degree cervical descent. She wishes to conserve her ovaries. What is the best treatment?

A. Abdominal hysterectomy
B. Vaginal hysterectomy
C. Uterine artery embolization
D. OC PILLS

5. Which surgical procedure has the highest incidence of ureteric injury?
   A. Vaginal hysterectomy
   B. Abdominal hysterectomy
   C. Weitheim's hysterectomy
   D. Anterior colporrhaphy

6. Most common complication of hysterectomy:
   A. Infection
   B. Bleeding
   C. GU injury
   D. VTE

7. Indications of vaginal hysterectomy:
   A. Prolapse
   B. Uterine size less than 12 weeks
   C. Adenomyosis
   D. All of the above

8. The most common presentation of vault prolapse:
   A. Bulge in vagina
   B. Sexual dysfunction
   C. Voiding difficulties
   D. Stress incontinence

9. Which is the preventive technique for posthysterectomy vault prolapse?
   A. Obliteration of pouch of Douglas
   B. Suturing the cardinal and uterosacral ligaments to the vaginal cuff at the time of abdominal hysterectomy
   C. Sacrospinous fixation (SSF) when the vault does not descend up to introitus
   D. Subtotal hysterectomy

10. Injury to ureter occurs most commonly at:
    A. Clamping infundibular ligament
    B. Clamping round ligament
    C. Clamping uterines
    D. Suturing the vault

11. Type 1 hysterectomy is:
    A. Simple extrafascial
    B. Wertheim's hysterectomy
    C. Radical hysterectomy
    D. Intrafascial

12. Which of the following factors are considered to choose route of hysterectomy in AUB cases?
    A. Safety
    B. Cost effectiveness
    C. Associated pathologies
    D. Surgeon's skill
    E. All of the above

13. In a case of postmenopausal bleeding if USG shows suspected polyp or thickened endometrium ideal option for the further workup before a decision of hysterectomy is made:
    A. Hysteroscopic targeted biopsy
    B. Dilatation and curettage
    C. Endometrial biopsy
    D. None of the above

14. What is the rationale of choosing a hysterectomy in a case of AUB? Choose the incorrect option:
    A. Failure of medical line of management
    B. Patient demands hysterectomy
    C. Failure following other modalities like TCRE, Balloon thermal ablation, etc.
    D. Compliance for follow-up unlikely
    E. Associated pathologies requiring surgical intervention
    F. Premalignant endometrial pathologies

15. Commonest uterine pathology which can be found in a patient operated for AUB?
    A. Adenomyosis
    B. Leiomyoma
    C. Polyps
    D. Endometrial hyperplasia

Answer Key

1. C	4. B	7. D	10. C	13. A
2. D	5. C	8. A	11. A	14. B
3. A	6. A	9. C	12. E	15. A

Reference

15. **A.** Rizvi G, Pandey H, Pant H, Chufal SS, Pant P (2013). Histopathological correlation of adenomyosis and leiomyoma in hysterectomy specimens as the cause of abnormal uterine bleeding in women in different age groups in the Kumaon region: A retroprospective study. *Journal of Mid-Life Health*, 4(1), 27–30. http://doi.org/10.4103/0976-7800.109631

Oophorectomy to Do or Not to Do

◘ *Suvarna Khadilkar*

1. Ovaries beyond menopause:
   A. Have no role to play
   B. Retain some reproductive function
   C. Continue to be an endocrine organ
   D. None of the above

2. Serum E2 levels after surgical menopause:
   A. < 10pg /ml
   B. < 25pg/ml
   C. ~50pg /ml
   D. None of the above

3. Choose the correct option about surgical menopause:
   A. Rapid drop of both estradiol and testosterone
   B. Testosterone supplements, most needed if still premenopausal at surgery
   C. MHT dosages need to be higher
   D. All of the above

4. Match the types of oophorectomy with its description:
   I. Opportunistic oophorectomy
   II. Interventional oophorectomy
   III. Prophylactic oophorectomy
   IV. Therapeutic oophorectomy
   V. Risk reducing oophorectomy
   A. Removal of healthy ovaries
   B. Opphorectomy in women at high risk of developing cancer
   C. Opphorectomy at the time of some other surgery
   D. Opphorectomy with a specific indication and recommendation
   E. Removal of diseased ovary

5. If the ovaries are normal, the chance of cancer later in life appears to be around:
   A. 12%
   B. 0.25%
   C. Nil
   D. 0.50%

6. All of the following statements are true except:
   A. Removal of the fallopian tubes and ovaries in women with the BRCA1 or BRCA2 gene mutation reduces the risk of ovarian cancer by 80%
   B. Primary peritoneal cancer can occur after prophylactic oophorectomy in BRCA1 and 2 positive patients
   C. Oophorectomy should be done routinely at hysterectomy for benign indications after the age of 50

D. Prophylactic oophorectomy in BRCA1 and 2 positive women protects them from ERPR positive breast cancer

7. A 40 years old lady underwent right sided radical mastectomy followed by complete course of chemotherapy. She was a case of infertility with PCOS conceived after 4 cycles of IUI with ovulation induction at the age of 34 and had 1 FTLSCS. BRACa1/2 status unknown but Ca breast was ER PR positive. She is getting infrequent cycles every 2–3 months bleeds for 3–4 days. There is no family history of Ca breast or any other cancer.

A. Bilateral prophylactic oophorectomy should be advised

B. Bilateral salpingectomy should be advised

C. Left sided mastectomy should be advised

D. A and B should be advised

8. 43 years old female c/o polymenorrhagia since 6–8 months. She wants to undergo hysterectomy in view of USG report: Uterus slightly bulky with two 0.5 cm fibroids in the body of uterus right side, ET 6 mm, ovaries normal, no other abnormalities

PR MH: 6–7days/20–24 days irregular, no dysmenorrhea, heavy flow with clots+

PAST MH occasional h/o of menorrhagia

OH: 3 FTLSCS bilateral TL done with last C-section 10 years back

No h/o malignancy in the family or any other major illness in past

O/E: PS healthy PV uterus RV parous mobility restricted FX clear

I. What would you do as a first step?

A. Hysterectomy

B. Endometrial sampling

C. Curettage

D. None of the above

II. If hysterectomy opted by the patient

A. Remove healthy ovaries at hysterectomy

B. Remove ovaries only if diseased

C. Remove one ovary

D. None of the above

9. State true or false:

A. If a woman is not at high-risk for ovarian cancer, keeping their ovaries might benefit her overall health and survival

B. All cause mortality after oophorectomies performed before age 50 will increase by approximately 10%

C. Younger the age at oophorectomy, lower is the risk of ischaemic heart disease

D. There is a 50% increase in dementia risk in oophorectomized women

E. Risks of Parkinson disease and anxiety or depression are unaltered if oophorectomy is done at younger age

F. Postmenopausal women with intact ovaries have less osteoporotic fractures than those who have undergone oophorectomy

G. Healthy ovaries must be retained till age of 65 at hysterectomy irrespective of indication for hysterectomy

10. Oophorectomies of healthy ovaries should be done at hysterectomy:

A. When women is premenopausal age

B. Up to 10 years of postmenopausal age

C. After 10 years of menopause or beyond age of 65

D. Both B and C are correct

Answer Key

1. C	7. D
2. A	8. I B
3. D	II B
4. I C	9. A True
II D	B True
III A	C False
IV E	D True
V B	E False
5. B	F True
6. C	G False
	10. C

Explanations and References

5. **B** Finch A, Beiner M, Lubinski J, et al. JAMA 2006 Hereditary Ovarian Cancer Clinical Study Group.

6. **C** Healthy ovaries should not be removed up to the age of 65 years key enzymes, CYP 19 A1 (Aromatase) and HSD17β1 show steroidogenic activity in the ovaries of postmenopausal women. At 2, 5, 10 years. Steroidogenic activity decreases but significant fall only 10 years after menopause.

    Brodowska A, Brodowski J, Laszczy ska M, Słuczanowska-Głbowska S, Rumianowski B, Rotter I, Starczewski A, Ratajczak MZ. Immunoexpression of aromatase cytochrome P450 and 17β-hydroxysteroid dehydrogenase in women's ovaries after menopause. *Journal of ovarian research*. 2014 Dec; 7(1):52.

7. **D** Bilateral prophylactic Oophorectomy and Bilateral Salpingectomy should be advised.

    There is good evidence that ER PR positive cancers are benefitted by oophorectomy. Also salpingectomy is known to prevent epithelial ovarian cancer she has hyperestrogenemia, so other breast will be also at risk so oophorectomy will take care of it. Mastectomy decision should be an individualized decision.

9.   Parker WH, Broder MS, Liu Z, et al. *Clin Obstet Gynecol*. 2007 Jun; 50(2):354–61.

10. **C** Authors did not demonstrate a survival benefit after oophorectomy at any age because the risks and benefits approximate each other after age 65.

    Parker WH, Broder MS, Liu Z, Shoupe D, Farquhar C, Berek JS. Ovarian conservation at the time of hysterectomy for benign disease. Obstetrics & Gynecology. 2005 Aug 1;106(2):219–26.

Chapter 45

Overactive Bladder

☑ *Suvarna Khadilkar*

1. What is overactive bladder?
   - **A.** It is a condition in which the bladder contracts involuntarily in response to filling
   - **B.** Symptoms of urgency, frequency, and nocturia with or without urge incontinence
   - **C.** Both A and B define overactive bladder
   - **D.** None of the above

2. Which of the three pictures given below depicts stress incontinence?
   - **A.** A
   - **B.** B

   - **C.** C
   - **D.** None

3. Which of the three pictures given below depicts urge incontinence?
   - **A.** A
   - **B.** B
   - **C.** C
   - **D.** None

4. Which of the three pictures given below depicts mixed incontinence?
   - **A.** A
   - **B.** B
   - **C.** C
   - **D.** None

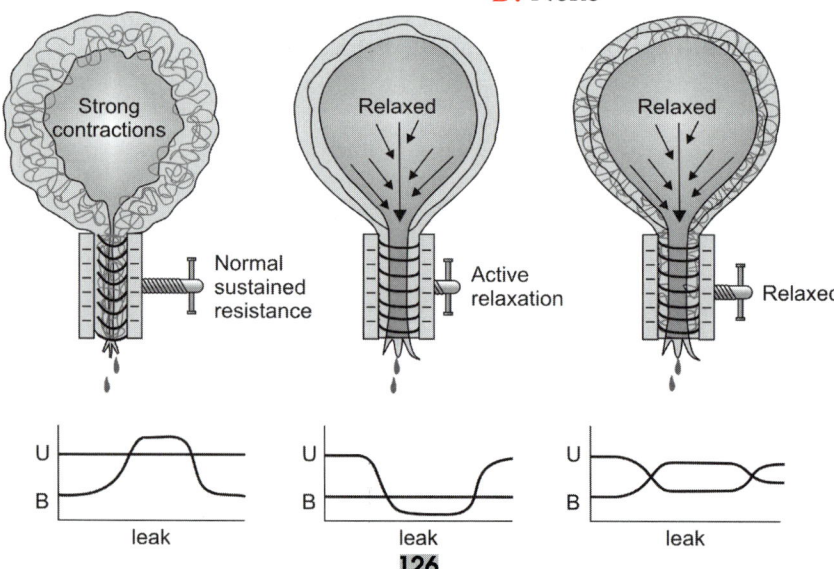

126

5. State True or False: Role of urodynamic studies in the diagnostic evaluation of bladder dysfunction:
   A. Urodynamic studies are indicated in all cases with genuine SUI
   B. It should be used selectively as it is an invasive procedure
   C. Studies are unable to identify hypereflexic bladder and involuntary contractions
   D. Urodynamic studies are indicated in cases with mixed aetiology

6. Menopause affects bladder function by all of the following mechanisms except:
   A. A reduced urinary flow rate
   B. Decreased urinary residual volume
   C. Reduced bladder capacity
   D. Lower maximal voiding pressures
   E. Decrease urethral pressure

7. Match the anticholinergic drugs used for overactive bladder and their dosages:
   1. Oxybutynin
   2. Tolterodine
   3. Solifenacin
   4. Darifenacin
   A. 5–10 mg once a day
   B. 7.5 or 15 mg extended release once a day
   C. 2 mg twice a day or 4 mg extended release once a day
   D. 5 mg maximum up to 4 times a day or 1.3, 2.6 or 3.9 patches used twice / week or intrarectal 5 mg BD

Answer Key

1. C	4. C	6. B
2. B	5. A. False	7. 1. D
3. A	B. True	2. C
	C. False	3. A
	D. True	4. B

Urinary Incontinence

☑ *Seema Sharma*

1. Which of the following urinary incontinence type does not require surgery?
   A. Urge incontinence
   B. Stress urinary incontinence
   C. Mixed urinary incontinence
   D. All of the above

2. In perimenopause which type of incontinence is more common:
   A. Urge incontinence
   B. True incontinence
   C. Stress incontinence (SUI)
   D. All of the above

3. All of the following about TVT used for SUI are true except:
   A. TVT is an acronym for transvaginal tape
   B. They are made of prolene polypropylene mesh
   C. They restore and reinforce the pubourethral ligaments at the midurethra and the suburethral vaginal hammock at the midurethra

   D. Indicated in urethral hypermobility or intrinsic sphincter deficiency (ISD)

4. How does hysterectomy affect SUI?
   A. Worsens
   B. Improves
   C. Does not affect
   D. NIL

5. Which of the following is true:
   A. Cystoscopy is a must after TOT sling insertion
   B. Duloxetine is highly effective in management of SUI
   C. A trial of antimuscarinics must be given to a patient of mixed incontinence before offering surgical management
   D. Mini slings are definitively better then full-length TOT sling

6. Most frequent complication of TVT is:
   A. Ureteric injury
   B. Bladder perforation
   C. Retropubic haematoma
   D. Injury to neurovascular bundle

Answer Key

| 1. A | 2. C | 3. A | 4. A | 5. C | 6. B |

Explanation

3. **A** TVT is tension free vaginal tape, TOT is trans obturator tape

Chapter 47

Genital Prolapse

◨ *Seema Sharma*

1. In postmenopausal women, following type of genital prolapse occurs:
   - A. Supravaginal elongation
   - B. Infravaginal elongation
   - C. General or total prolapse
   - D. All of the above

2. The prevalence of pelvic organ prolapse (POP) in women over 40 years of age, based solely on patients symptoms ranges from:
   - A. 8 to 18%
   - B. 0.9 to 3.9%
   - C. 2.9 to 8%
   - D. 18.3 to 22.3%

3. According to recent estimates life-time risk of women undergoing surgery for pelvic organ prolapse or stress incontinence is:
   - A. 10%
   - B. 20%
   - C. 30%
   - D. 40%

4. Likelihood of reoperation for recurrence after primary pelvic reconstruction surgery in present context is:
   - A. 1.6 – 4.6%
   - B. 5.6 – 13%
   - C. 13 – 17%
   - D. 15 – 20%

5. All of the following are high-risk factors for pelvic organ prolapse except:
   - A. Familial and genetic linkage
   - B. Smoking
   - C. Nulliparity
   - D. Menopause

6. Currently the most commonly used reconstructive material in surgical augmented repair of pelvic organ prolapse is:
   - A. Polypropylene
   - B. Polyethylene
   - C. Polytetrafluroethylene
   - D. Polyglactin 910

7. According to FDA the transvaginal meshes are now classified is:
   - A. Class I
   - B. Class II
   - C. Class III
   - D. Post amendments devices

8. Xenografts used in POP surgery as augmenting material are:
   - A. Acellular extracts of collagen harvested from other non-human species and processed to be used in humans
   - B. Harvested from cadaveric fascia of human donors

C. Harvested from and then implanted in same patient

D. Having no risk of rejection and infection

9. The use of autografts for POP repair is limited by all of the following factors except:
   A. Morbidity at the harvest site
   B. No risk of host immune response
   C. Inconsistent quantity and quality of the harvested anaterial
   D. Increased operative time and blood loss for procurement

10. Woven meshes as augmenting materials used in POP surgery are associated with:
    A. Higher complication rates
    B. More porous than knitted mashes
    C. More flexible than knitted mashes
    D. More favourable host immune response

11. Pick out the right statement:
    A. POP is not always chronic and progressive. Spontaneous regression is common, especially for grade 1 prolapse
    B. POP is always progressive and surgery is the only answer
    C. POP in postmenopausal women occurs due to lack of progesterone in the body for long-time
    D. Kegels exercises are not useful in POP at menopause

12. If a genital prolapse of procidentia type is seen beyond menopause in otherwise a low-risk patient:
    A. Estrogen vaginal cream can cure it
    B. Estriol cream should not be used preoperatively
    C. Estriol cream used preoperatively improves surgical success and healing
    D. Colpocleisis is the only option

Answer Key

| 1. C | 3. B | 5. C | 7. C | 9. B | 11. A |
| 2. C | 4. B | 6. A | 8. A | 10. A | 12. C |

References

2. Climacteric, 2017; Vol 20 No. 6 (510–517)
3. Climacteric, 2017; Vol 20 No. 6 (510–517)
4. Climacteric, 2017; Vol 20 No. 6 (510–517)
11. Handa VL, Garrett E, Hendrix S, Gold E, Robbins J. Progression and remission of pelvic organ prolapse: a longitudinal study of menopausal women. *American Journal of Obstetrics and Gynecology.* 2004 Jan 1; 190(1):27–32.

Genital Atrophy

☑ *Preeti Deshpande*

1. The term atrophic vaginitis has been replaced by:
   A. Vulvovaginal atrophy
   B. Genitourinary syndrome of menopause
   C. Postmenopausal syndrome
   D. Menopausal atrophy

2. The term genitourinary syndrome of menopause includes:
   A. Genital symptoms
   B. Sexual symptoms
   C. Urinary symptoms
   D. All of the above

3. Estrogen receptors are present on:
   A. Vagina
   B. Vulva
   C. Pelvic fascia and musculature
   D. All of the above

4. What changes occur after menopause?
   A. Vaginal pH increases
   B. Vaginal flora changes
   C. Epithelium becomes thinner
   D. Collagen content reduces
   E. All of the above

5. Estrogen stimulation does all of the following except:
   A. Maintains the collagen content of epithelium, which affects its thickness and elasticity
   B. Maintains acid mucopolysaccharides and hyaluronic acid, which keeps epithelial surfaces moist
   C. Maintains optimal genital blood flow
   D. Maintains the alkaline pH

6. Which one of the following is responsible for acidic pH of vagina (3.5 to 5) in premenopausal women?
   A. Estrogen
   B. Glycogen content of sloughed cells of vaginal epithelium
   C. Doderlein's bacilli
   D. All of the above

7. Classic vaginal findings of atrophy include all except:
   A. Pale, dry vaginal epithelium
   B. Polypoidal vagina
   C. Smooth and shiny with loss of rugosity
   D. The vaginal fornices become obliterated

8. State true or false:
   A. Genitourinary syndrome may lead to genital prolapse
   B. Symptomatic vaginal atrophy occurs in about 40% of menopausal women
   C. Laboratory tests are always necessary for diagnosis

D. Treatment to be started when symptoms cause her distress and hamper her day-to-day life

E. First line of treatment is through vaginal moisturisers and lubricants for dryness of vagina

F. Gold standard therapy—low dose vaginal estrogen creams and progesterone therapy

G. Safety data of vaginal estrogen is available only up to one year of use

Answer Key

1. B	4. E	7. B	C False	F False
2. D	5. D	8. A True	D True	G True
3. D	6. D	B True	E True	

Explanation and Reference

1. **B** The terms vulvovaginal atrophy (VVA) and atrophic vaginitis is not adequate for describing the range of menopausal symptoms associated with physical changes of the vulva, vagina, and lower urinary tract associated with estrogen deficiency. VVA describes the appearance of the postmenopausal vulva and vagina without specifying the presence of associated symptoms. So new term genitourinary syndrome was recommended by International Society for the Study of Women's Sexual Health and The North American Menopause Society at terminology consensus conference 2014.

Portman DJ, Gass ML. (2014). Genitourinary syndrome of menopause: New terminology for vulvovaginal atrophy. J Sex Med, 11: 2865–72. doi:10.1111/jsm.12686

Perimenopausal Bleeding and Case Scenarios

☑ *Deepali Prakash Kale*

1. 52 years postmenopausal female with ultrasonography suggestive of endomterial thickness of 8 mm. The cut-off endometrial thickness for postmenopausal female is:
   A. 6 mm
   B. 4 mm
   C. 8 mm
   D. 10 mm

2. The incidence of carcinoma endometrium in endometrial polyp is:
   A. 10%
   B. <5%
   C. 1%
   D. 20%

3. The chances of progress to carcinoma in endometrial hyperplasia without atypia over 20 years period is:
   A. 1%
   B. 5%
   C. 1%
   D. 20%

4. The first line treatment of endometrial hyperplasia without atypia in a 46-year-old female is:
   A. LNG-IUS
   B. Medroxyprogesterone acetate
   C. Continuous norethisterone
   D. Combined oral contraceptives

5. The duration of treatment for conservative management of endometrial hyperplasia without atypia before next surveillance is:
   A. 1 month
   B. 3 months
   C. 6 months
   D. 1 year

6. Endometrial surveillance interval in case of endometrial hyperplasia without atypia is:
   A. 2 negative biopsies 6 monthly
   B. 4 negative biopsies 6 monthly
   C. 6 negative 1 yearly interval

7. First investigation to rule out endometrial hyperplasia in a 55 years old female with postmenopausal bleeding is:
   A. Transvaginal sonography
   B. Dilatation and curretage
   C. Hysteroscopy guided biopsy
   D. MRI

8. In women who want to conserve uterus, routine endometrial surveillance in endometrial hyperplasia with atypia is:
   A. 3 monthly till 2 consecutive negative biopsies
   B. 1 monthy till 3 negative biopsies

C. 6 monthly till 4 negative biopsies

D. 1 yearly till 3 negative biopsies

9. 54-year-old woman presents after one episode of postmenopausal bleeding. She is on tamoxifen for her breast malignancy. The side effects of tamoxifen are:
   A. Mood swings
   B. Hot flushes
   C. Endometrial hyperplasia
   D. All A, B, C are correct

10. 52 years old female with history of Ca breast on treatment with tamoxifen c/o heavy menstrual bleeding. Best suitable option for her is:
    A. Stop tamoxifen
    B. Consult oncologist and reassess the need for tamoxifen
    C. Endometrial biopsy every 6 months
    D. Hysterectomy

11. Endometrial hyperplasia confined to endometrial polyp is managed as:
    A. Hysteroscopic polypectomy
    B. Endometrial biopsy
    C. Both A and B
    D. Endometrial ablation and polypectomy

12. Risk factor for endometrial hyperplasia are all except:
    A. BMI 38 kg/m^2
    B. Combined HRT
    C. Anovulation at the time of menopause
    D. PCOS

13. Most common endometrial histopathological finding associated with granulosa cell tumours is:
    A. Proliferative endometrium
    B. Atrophic endometrium
    C. Hyperplastic endometrium
    D. Adenocarcinoma

14. The rate of need for repeat procedure after uterine artery emobilisation in women older than 45 years is:
    A. <25%

B. 50%

C. 70%

D. 40 %

15. True about endometrial polyps is:
    A. They are common in <20 years age group
    B. Can be asymptomatic or may cause heavy menstrual bleeding.
    C. In both pre and postmenopausal women they loose their apoptotic regulation and overexpress estrogen and progesterone receptors
    D. There is no role of conservative management

16. Medical management of fibroids is best indicated in a fibroid:
    A. <3 cm, distorting the cavity, asymptomatic
    B. >3 cm distorting the cavity asymptomatic
    C. <3 cm not distorting the cavity causing heavy menstrual bleeding
    D. None of the above

17. A 57-year-old woman presents after two episodes of postmenoapsual bleeding next step in her management should be:
    A. Wait and watch
    B. Hysterectomy
    C. Rule out malignancy
    D. None of the above

18. The sensitivity of pipelle sample for detection of endometrial cancer is:
    A. 96%
    B. 45%
    C. 30%
    D. 10%

19. 65-year-old female presents with postmenopausal bleeding and the ovarian cystic enlargement on ultrasonography. Which is the most likely associated ovarian pathology in this condition?
    A. Serous cystadenoma
    B. Mucinous cystadenoma

C. Granulosa cell tumor

D. Dermoid cyst

20. The known side effect of drug tamoxifen is endometrial hyperplasia. This drug belongs to following class:

A. ACE inhibitor

B. Dopamine agonist

C. Progesterone antagonist

D. Selective oestrogen receptor modulator

21. In cases of perimenopausal abnor-mal uterine bleeding if the uterus is normal

on examination, the most appropriate method of biopsy is:

A. Office endometrial aspiration

B. In hospital dilatation and curettage

C. Fractional curettage

D. Colposcopically directed biopsy

22. Which is the most common cause of perimenopausal bleeding?

A. Endometrial atrophy

B. Endometrial hyperplasia

C. Endometrial polyp

D. Cancer endometrium

Answer Key

1. B	5. C	9. A	13. C	17. D	21. A
2. A	6. A	10. B	14. A	18. A	22. A
3. B	7. A	11. C	15. C	19. C	
4. A	8. A	12. B	16. C	20. D	

Explanations and References

1-22 Source: Green-top Guideline No. 67 RCOG/BSGE Joint Guideline I February 2016.

4. **A** The LNG-IUS should be the first-line medical treatment because compared with oral progestogens it has a higher disease regression rate with a more favorable bleeding profile and it is associated with fewer adverse effects. Continuous progestogens should be used (medroxyprogesterone 10–20 mg/day or norethisterone10–15 mg/day for women who decline the LNG-IUS. The LNG-IUS achieves a higher concentration of levonorgestrel at the level of the endometrium compared with oral progestogens:
   Ioannis D Gallos, et al. Oral progestogens vs levonorgestrel-releasing intrauterine system for endometrial hyperplasia: a systematic review and meta-analysis, American Journal of *Obstetrics and Gynecology,* Volume 203, Issue 6, December 2010, 547.e1-547.e10.

5. **C** Endometrial surveillance should be done at 6-monthly intervals.

6. **A** At least two consecutive 6-monthly negative biopsies should be obtained prior to the cure. The women with the disease relapse may present with abnormal vaginal bleeding and advised to seek a further referral. In women at higher risk of relapse, such as women with a BMI of 35 or greater or those treated with oral progestogens, 6-monthly endometrial biopsies are recommended. Once two consecutive negative endometrial biopsies have been obtained then long-term follow-up should be considered with annual endometrial biopsies.

13. **C** Evans AJ III, et al. Clinicopathological review of 118 granulosa and 82 theca cell tumors. *Obstet Gynecol* 55:213, 1980.

14. **A** Review Pregnancy outcomes after uterine artery embolization for fibroids. The obstetrician and gynaecologists: 2009; 11:265–70.

16. **C** Vikram Sinai Talaulikar. Medical therapy for fibroids: An overview, Best Practice & Research Clinical Obstetrics & Gynaecology, Volume 46, January 2018, Pages 48–56.

18. **A** Clark TJ, Mann CH, Shah N, Khan KS, Song F, Gupta JK. Accuracy of outpatient endometrial biopsy in the diagnosis of endometrial cancer: a systematic quantitative review. BJOG 2002;109:313–21.

Case Scenarios: Stress Urine Incontinence/Urge Incontinence

◙ *Preeti Deshpande and Suvarna Khadilkar*

1. A 56 years old lady presented with passage of urine on coughing and laughing. Urine routine examination was normal. Most likely diagnosis is:
   A. Overactive bladder
   B. Stress urinary incontinence
   C. Urge incontinence
   D. None of the above

2. A 60 years old lady presented with urgency to micturate. She was unable to reach the toilet at times. A urine routine was normal. This is a case of:
   A. Overactive bladder
   B. Stress urinary incontinence
   C. Urge incontinence
   D. None of the above

3. A 55-year-old lady came with complaints of dyspaurenia and vaginal dryness. She had episodes of recurrent urinary tract infection. The last episode was treated 3 months back. The correct line of treatment is:
   A. Darifenacin
   B. USG for residual urine

C. Vaginal estrogen cream
D. Both B and C are correct

4. A 59 years old lady presented with urinary tract infection. Her urine routine showed 50 pus cells per high power field. Her urine culture was awaited. She had frequency and urgency to pass urine. Her immediate treatment will include:
   A. Empiric followed by specific antibiotic as per urine culture sensitivity
   B. Menopause hormone therapy
   C. Oxybutynin
   D. None of the above

5. A 60 years old lady presented with poor bone mineral density (T score –2,5) on investigation and body pain. She had a fall on rushing for urgency to pass urine. She needs to be protected from the risk of fractures.
   A. Biophosphonates can be used
   B. Darifenacin is ideal drug
   C. Menopause hormone therapy
   D. Both A and B may be required

Answer Key

| 1. B | 2. C | 3. D | 4. A | 5. D |

Explanations

3. **D** Both USG for residual urine and vaginal estrogen cream are correct. Recurrent urinary infection may be due to large amount of residual urine which acts as a reservoir for harboring infection so after ruling out that treatment with local estrogens will improve atrophic changes and reduce the number of attacks of recurrent Infections. Large residual urine indicates a cystocele or other neurological causes which would need specific treatment.

4. **A** Her immediate problem is acute infection and needs to be treated with antibiotic.

5. **D** As she is 60 years old MHT is contraindicated in her. Raloxifene 60 mg can be used but does not reduce the risk of non-vertebral fractures. So bisphosphonates is drug of choice. Darifenacin is drug suitable to tackle her overactive bladder hence both A & B are correct.

Case Scenarios: Genital Prolapse

☐ *Seema Sharma*

CASE 1: A 57 years old postmenopausal woman Para–8 all full term vaginal home deliveries presented in gynae outpatient clinic, with complaint of something descending through vagina since 3 years, spotting P/V on and off since 2 months. On examination whole of her uterus was lying outside with complete eversion of vagina. She is had no other medical illness in past. Answer the following:

1. What is the most probable cause for spotting per vaginum in this case?
   A. Cervical cancer
   B. Decubitus ulcer
   C. Blood dyscrasias
   D. Endometrial cancer

2. Most effective treatment for her is:
   A. Pessary
   B. Lefort colpocleisis
   C. Vaginal hysterectomy (VH) with vault repair
   D. Diet and lifestyle changes

3. Regarding classification of prolapse for uterine descent which is not correct?
   A. First degree descent implies that the cervix descends below its normal level on straining but does not protrude from the vulva
   B. First degree descent implies that the cervix descends below its normal level on straining and protrudes from the vulva
   C. Second degree descent implies that the cervix reaches up to the vulva on straining
   D. Procidentia means whole of the uterus is prolapsed outside the vulva

4. Which of the following are etiologies of uterovaginal prolapse:
   A. Aging
   B. Estrogen deprivation
   C. Intrinsic collagen abnormalities
   D. Chronic increase in intraabdominal pressure
   E. Acute and chronic trauma of vaginal delivery
   F. All of above

5. Following is not a posterior vaginal wall defect:
   A. Enterocele
   B. Rectocele
   C. Perineal body descent
   D. Perineal tear

CASE 2: A 48 years old woman P2 both cesarean sections presented with mass descending down the vagina on exami-nation leading edge is + 1 cm.

6. According to POP-Q she falls in:
   A. Stage 0
   B. Stage II
   C. Stage I
   D. Stage III

7. Which of the following statements is false regarding the examination of a patient with prolapse?
   A. The maximal extent of prolapse is demonstrated with a standing straining examination when the bladder is empty
   B. Resting tone and voluntary contraction of the anal sphincters should be assessed during rectovaginal examination
   C. Women with prolapse and urinary incontinence should have stress testing performed with the prolapse reduction because this will mimic bladder and urethral function when the prolapse is treated
   D. Screening for presence of UTI or CIN is not needed at the time of examination

8. Most appropriate treatment for her at this age would be:
   A. Sling surgery
   B. Pessary
   C. VH with lateral window technique (to avoid bladder injury)
   D. Kegel's exercises

9. All of the following are true supports of the uterus except:
   A. Mackenrodt's ligaments
   B. Uterosacral ligaments
   C. Broad ligament
   D. Pubocervical fascia
   E. Rectovaginal fascia

10. Following are the first level of support in DeLancy system:
    A. Cardinal ligament

B. Pubocervical fascia
C. Rectovaginal fascia
D. Pubourethral ligaments
E. Perineal body

CASE 3: A 75 years old postmenopausal female presented with 2° U-V prolapse. She gives history of spotting and has severe COPD. She is currently on anti-hypertensives since 15 years and gives family history of HTN and MI she also gives history of fracture at right hip joint 2 years back with deformity in right leg. Answer the following for her:

11. Suitable option for her management:
    A. Pessary
    B. VH with colpoperineorrhaphy
    C. Sling operation
    D. LAVH with colpoperineorrhaphy

12. Which of the following is not an indication for use of pessary:
    A. When future childbearing is intended in near future
    B. Refusal for operation by patient
    C. As a therapeutic test
    D. Prolapse with pregnancy
    E. Non-healing decubitus ulcer

13. All of the following are complications associated with pessary except:
    A. Bacterial vaginitis, ulceration of vaginal wall
    B. Cervicitis
    C. Carcinoma of vaginal wall
    D. Impaction of pessary
    E. Reduction of prolapse
    F. Strangulation of prolapsed tissue

14. Following are true for management of prolapse except:
    A. Any decision for surgical intervention should take account of how prolapse is affecting lifestyle
    B. Vaginal pessary can be used in elderly patients with prolapse with associated medical complications which contradict surgery

C. Vaginal hysterectomy is the only treatment of prolapse in all women
D. Sling surgeries are indicated in women desiring to retain reproductive function

E. Assessment of SUI is must during examination of prolapse so that the same can be corrected during surgery

Answer Key

1. B	4. F	7. D	10. A	13. E
2. C	5. A	8. C	11. A	14. C
3. B	6. B	9. C	12. E	

Explanations and References

5. **A** Delancey support levels
   - **Level 1:** The cardinal-uterosacral ligament complex provides apical attachment of the uterus and vaginal vault to the bony sacrum. Uterine prolapse occurs when the cardinal-uterosacral ligament complex breaks or is attenuated.
   - **Level 2:** The arcus tendineous fascia pelvis and the fascia overlying the levator ani muscles provide support to the middle part of the vagina.
   - **Level 3:** The urogenital diaphragm and the perineal body provide support to the lower part of the vagina.

   DeLancey JO. Anatomic aspects of vaginal eversion after hysterectomy. *Am J Obstet Gynecol* 1992; 166:1717–24. [PubMed Barber MD. Contemporary views on female pelvic anatomy. *Cleve Clin J Med* 2005; 72(suppl 4):S3–11.[PubMed]

6. **B** Pelvic organ prolapse quantification system. This system defines the extent of prolapse by measuring the descent of anterior, posterior, and apical segments of the vaginal wall relative to the vaginal hymen.
   - **Stage 0:** No prolapse
   - **Stage I:** The most distal portion of the prolapse is > 1 cm above the level of the hymen
   - **Stage II:** The most distal portion of the prolapse is ≤ 1 cm proximal or distal to the hymen
   - **Stage III:** The most distal portion of the prolapse is > 1 cm below the hymen but protrudes no further than 2 cm less than the total length of the vagina
   - **Stage IV:** Complete eversion of the vagina.

   Hall AF, Theofrastous JP, Cundiff GW, Harris RL, Hamilton LF, Swift SE, et al. Interobserver and intraobserver reliability of the proposed International Continence Society, Society of Gynecologic Surgeons, and American Urogynecologic Society pelvic organ prolapse classification system. *Am J Obstet Gynecol* 1996; 175:1467–70.

Path Breaking Trials

☑ *Meeta and Suvarna Khadilkar*

1. The hypothesis of 'window of opportunity' developed after:
   A. WHI
   B. ELITE
   C. Nurses health study
   D. KEEPS

2. The hypothesis of 'window of opportunity' for HT use may be applicable to:
   A. Coronary heart disease
   B. Alzheimer disease
   C. A and B
   D. Colon cancer

3. The objective of early versus late intervention trial with estradiol (ELITE) was:
   A. To test the cardiovascular effects of postmenopausal hormone therapy with the timing of therapy initiation
   B. To assess the effect of oral versus transdermal estrogen on cardiovascular parameters
   C. To assess the benefit on quality of life
   D. All the above

4. The women in ELITE trial were offered?
   A. 17β estradiol and dydrogesterone

   B. 17β estradiol and medroxyprogesterone
   C. 17β estradiol and norethisterone
   D. 17β estradiol and progesterone gel

5. The Danish osteoporosis prevention study:
   A. Is a prospective multicentre trial evaluating the effect of hormone replacement therapy as primary prevention of osteoporotic fractures in healthy women treated early in postmenopause. with 17-β-estradiol and norethisterone acetate
   B. The only study with a 10 years randomized intervention
   C. Planned duration was 20 years
   D. All are true

6. The Danish osteoporosis prevention study-select the right answer:
   A. Early initiation and prolonged hormone replacement therapy resulted in an increased risk of breast cancer or stroke in combined regime
   B. Early initiation and prolonged continuous combined hormone replacement therapy did not change the risk of the combined

endpoint of mortality, myocardial infarction, or heart failure
C. Women with surgical menopause receiving unopposed 17-β-estradiol, there was a significant reduction in breast cancer
D. A significant increase in fat mass and trunk fat has been observed in the treated group with hormone replacement therapy

7. The Kronos early estrogen prevention study (KEEPS) was done:
   A. To assess atherosclerosis progression and cardiovascular risk factors after HT initiation
   B. To assess the risk of the combined endpoint of mortality, myocardial infarction, or heart failure
   C. To assess the primary changes in bone mineral density
   D. To assess the primary prevention of fragility fractures

8. Which statement regarding the Kronos early estrogen prevention study (KEEPS), 2012 is true:
   A. An open label study
   B. There was a significant progression of atherosclerosis during 4 years of follow-up in healthy, recently menopausal women
   C. There was no excess of cases of venous thromboembolism
   D. Low dose transdermal estrogen with oral progesterone was used

9. First randomized trial to indicate that HT should not be used for secondary prevention of CVD was?
   A. WHI
   B. Women's estrogen lipid-lowering hormone atherosclerosis regression trial (WELL-HART)
   C. PEPI
   D. HERS

10. The first study to report the effect of HT on hot flashes in older post-menopausal women was?
    A. WHI
    B. HERS
    C. DOPS
    D. ELITE

11. Million women study was done in?
    A. USA
    B. UK
    C. Australia
    D. Denmark

12. True statement about million women study is:
    A. Insignificant increased risk of breast cancer was seen in the women on combined HRT (estrogen and progestogens) and less so with estrogen only and tibolone
    B. Women aged 50–75 years
    C. One to one interview
    D. Size of a study alone does not establish association of disease with intervention

13. The women's health initiative Which of the following statement is not true?
    A. Multi-center, double-blinded placebo-controlled primary prevention trial
    B. To assess long-term health outcomes fracture risk, heart disease and stroke
    C. To assess quality of life
    D. Average age 63 years

14. Which of the following statements about WHI is not true?
    A. Began in the 1990s
    B. Reported its main findings in 2002
    C. Trial ended after 5 years, was to run for 12 years
    D. Trial terminated after 5.8 years

15. Treatment arms in the WHI included:
    A. Combined estrogen conjugated equine estrogen, (CEE) plus progestin (medroxyprogesterone

acetate) (E + P), Estrogens only (CEE)
- **B.** Calcium and vitamin D
- **C.** Placebo
- **D.** All of the above

16. The major problem of WHI:
- **A.** Age of subjects
- **B.** HT to all regardless of symptoms
- **C.** Women did not represent the ideal candidates for common indication for HT
- **D.** All of the above

17. The initial reports of the WHI results of treatment with E+P versus placebo were most significant for the demonstration of increased absolute risk:
- **A.** Of venous thromboembolism, coronary events, stroke, and the diagnosis of breast cancer
- **B.** Of the increased risk of invasive breast cancer
- **C.** Of no effect on fragility fractures
- **D.** Failure to demonstrate an overall health benefit

18. WHI in the ET group in women age 50–59 years, statistically confirmed a decreased risk in all except:
- **A.** Of total deaths
- **B.** Of coronary heart disease
- **C.** In breast cancer diagnosis
- **D.** In venous thromboembolism

19. Association of unopposed exogenous estrogen and endometrial carcinoma was found in?
- **A.** 1975
- **B.** 1985
- **C.** 1995
- **D.** None of the above

20. HT-induced prevention of hip fractures in population based study was demonstrated in?
- **A.** WHI
- **B.** Wisdom
- **C.** Nurses health study
- **D.** NORA

21. PEPI TRIAL:
- **A.** Studied the effect of estrogen-based HT on heart disease
- **B.** LDL is lowered, triglycerides are raised
- **C.** Progestogen interferes with the positive effect that estrogen has on LDL
- **D.** All are true

22. Lessons learnt from WHI:
- **A.** Pathophysiology of age-related benefits and risks of HT
- **B.** Differences on the effects of HT do not exist between various E+P and E regimes
- **C.** Analyses, interpretation and communication of results should be done promptly
- **D.** All of the above

23. Observational studies that compared the effect of oral versus transdermal estrogen therapy on VTE except:
- **A.** ESTHER
- **B.** SWAN
- **C.** E3N
- **D.** Million woman

24. False statement about venous thromboembolism (VT) in ESTHER study 2007 is:
- **A.** No increased risk with progesterone, micronized progesterone, and pregnane derivatives (including medroxyprogesterone acetate) no increased risk
- **B.** Increased risk up to four times with norethindrone, norpregnance derivates
- **C.** Transdermal HT presented minimal risk
- **D.** Oral HT risk was doubled

25. Nurses health study pick the false statement:
- **A.** Began in 1975, involved 121, 700 nurses
- **B.** It was an observational study

C. Aim was to study the effect of HT on heart disease.

D. Aim was to study the effects of long-term oral contraception use

26. Strengths of WHI include:
   A. Understanding of the timing hypothesis
   B. Use of HT for primary and secondary prevention of heart disease
   C. Understanding the effect on fragility fractures
   D. All of the above

27. HOPE—pick the false option:
   A. Prospective, RC double blind placebo controlled multicentric trial
   B. 2805 healthy PM women with intact uterus
   C. Age 40–75 years
   D. Aims was to study the effect of low dose HT on menopausal symptoms

28. In the studies involving raloxifene—pick the wrong statement:
   A. MORE trial was to designed to look at the effects on vertebral fractures

B. RUTH trial enrolled women with CVD
C. RUTH trial excluded women with CVD
D. STAR trial for chemoprotection for breast cancer

29. The THEBES study of tibolone—pick the right answer:
   A. Designed to study the histology of the endometrium and breast
   B. Designed to study the relation to endometrial and breast cancer
   C. Did show an increase in VTE
   D. Considered osteoporotic frac-tures as secondary end points

30. Tibolone and breast cancer—pick the right answer:
   A. Liberate trial was on women after breast cancer
   B. Lift trial showed a decreased risk of breast cancer
   C. Tibolone is preferable to conventional HT in women with mammography dense breasts
   D. All the above

Answer Key

1. A	7. A	13. C	19. A	25. C
2. C	8. C	14. C	20. A	26. D
3. A	9. D	15. D	21. D	27. C
4. D	10. B	16. D	22. A	28. C
5. D	11. B	17. C	23. B	29. A
6. C	12. A	18. D	24. D	30. D

Explanations and an account of trials on menopausal women:

Study	Type	Location	Dates	N	Ages; mean	Hormone formulation
WHI (E+P)	RCT	US	1993-2002	16608	50-79; 63	CE 0.625 mg MPA 2.5 mg
Intact uterus. Stopped early after 5.2 years (planned for 8); increased CHD events and invasive breast cancer.						
WHI (E)	RCT	US	1993-2004	10739	50-79; 63	CE 0.625 mg
Status: posthysterectomy. Stopped early after 6.8 years; Increased risk CVA:, stroke lack of CHD benefits.						
PEPI	RCT	US	1989-1994	875	45-64; 67	CE 0.625 mg ± MPA 10 mg (days 1-12) ± MPA 2.5 mg QD ± P4 200 mg (days 1-12)
Healthy women; 3 years follow-up. HT improved lipoprotein profiles. Unopposed estrogen associated with high rate endometrial hyperplasia.						
HERS	RCT	US	1993-1998	2763	67	CE 0.625 mg MPA 2.5 mg
Subjects had known CHD. HT 36 months.						
NHS	Obs				34-59	
SWAN	Obs	US	1996-current	3302	42-52	As per patient preference (including no HT)

Multiracial, multiethnic (Caucasian, African American, Hispanic, Chinese, Japanese); includes premenopausal; yearly visits—currently tracking 12th-13th visits. Following bone density, cardiovascular health, mood, symptoms.

MWS	Obs	UK	1996-current	1084110	50-64; 56	As per patient preference
WISDOM	RCT	UK, Australia, New Zealand	1999-2002	5692	50-69; 63	CE 0.625 mg ± MPA 2.5 or 5 mg
Stopped early after median 12 months follow-up (planned 10 years) because of WHI results.						
ELITE	RCT	US	2004-2013	643	6 years vs. 10 years postmeno.	E2 1 mg PO
2.5 years planned; endpoint atherosclerosis by carotid ultrasoun d.						
KEEPS	RCT	US	2005-2012	727	42-58,52	CE 0.45 mg or E2 50 mcg transdermal P4 200 mg (days 1-12)
Harvard Mood	Obs	US	1995-2006	460	36-45	No RX
(DOPS) Schierback et al	RCT	Denmark	1990-2008	1006	49.7 ± 2.8	2 mg synthetic 17-β-estradiol for 12 days, 2 mg 17-β-estradiol plus 1 mg norethisterone acetate for 10 days, and 1 mg 17-β-estradiol for six days or 2 mg 17β estradiol for hysterectomized

References

Important pathbreaking trials in menopause and MHT:

1. Effects of hormone therapy on bone mineral density: results from the postmenopausal estrogen/progestin interventions (PEPI) trial. The Writing Group for the PEPI. *JAMA* 1996; 276:1389–96.

2. Grady D, Brown JS, Vittinghoff E, Applegate W, Varner E, Snyder T. HERS Research Group. Postmenopausal hormones and incontinence: the Heart and Estrogen/Progestin Replacement Study. *Obstet Gynecol* 2001; 97:116–20.

3. Writing Group for the Women's Health Initiative. Investigators risks and benefits of estrogen plus progestin in healthy postmenopausal women: principal results from the women's health initiative randomized controlled trial. JAMA. 2002; 288:321–33.

4. Anderson GL, Limacher M, Assaf AR, Bassford T, Beresford SA, Black H, et al. Women's Health Initiative Steering Committee. Effects of conjugated equine estrogen in postmenopausal women with hysterectomy: the Women's Health Initiative randomized controlled trial. *JAMA*. 2004; 291(14):1701–12.

5. Hulley S, Grady D, Bush T, Furberg C, Herrington D, Riggs B, Vittinghoff E. Randomized trial of estrogen plus progestin for secondary prevention of coronary heart disease in postmenopausal women. Heart and Estrogen/progestin Replacement Study (HERS) Research Group. *JAMA*. 1998; 280(7):605–13.

6. Rossouw JE, Prentice RL, Manson JE, et al. Postmenopausal hormone therapy and risk of cardiovascular disease by age and years since menopause. *JAMA*. 2007; 297(13):1465–77.

7. Renoux C, Suissa S. Hormone therapy administration in postmenopausal women and risk of stroke. Womens Health. 2011; 7(3):355–61.

8. Barrett-Connor E, Grady D, Sashegyi A, et al. MORE investigators (multiple outcomes of raloxifene evaluation). Raloxifene and cardiovascular events in osteoporotic postmenopausal women: four-year results from the MORE (multiple outcomes of raloxifene evaluation) randomized trial. *JAMA*. 2002; 287(7): 847–57.

9. Beral V. Million Women Study Collaborators, Bull D, Green J, et al. Ovarian cancer and hormone replacement therapy in the million women study. *Lancet*. 2007; 369(9574):1703–10.

10. Chlebowski RT, Kuller LH, Prentice RL, et al. WHI investigators breast cancer after use of estrogen plus progestin in postmenopausal women. *N Engl J Med*. 2009; 360(6):573–87.

11. Recker RR, Mitlak BH, Ni X, et al. Long-term raloxifene for postmenopausal osteoporosis. *Curr Med Res Opin*. 2011; 27(9): 1755–61.

12. Shumaker SA, Legault C, Kuller L, et al. Women's Health Initiative Memory Study. Conjugated equine estrogens and incidence of probable dementia and mild cognitive impairment in postmenopausal women: Women's Health Initiative Memory Study. *JAMA*. 2004; 291(24):2947–58.

13. Farquhar C, Marjoribanks J, Lethaby A, et al. Long term hormone therapy for perimenopausal and postmenopausal women. Cochrane Database Syst Rev. 2009; 15(2): CD004143.

14. Johnson JR, Lacey JV Jr, Lazovich D, et al. Menopausal hormone therapy and risk of colorectal cancer. Cancer Epidemiol Biomark Prev. 2009; 18(1):196–203.

15. Estrogen and progestogen use in peri- and postmenopausal women: March 2007 position statement of the North American Menopause Society. Menopause 2007; 14:1–17.

16. Pinkerton JA, Aguirre FS, Blake J, Cosman F, Hodis H, Hoffstetter S, Kaunitz AM, Kingsberg SA, Maki PM, Manson JA, Marchbanks P. The 2017 hormone therapy position statement of the North American Menopause Society. Menopause. 2017 Jul 1; 24(7):728–53.

17. Kenemans P, Bundred NJ, Foidart JM, Kubista E, von Schoultz B, Sismondi P, Vassilopoulou-Sellin R, Yip CH, Egberts J, Mol-Arts M, Mulder R. Safety and efficacy of tibolone in breast-cancer patients with vasomotor symptoms: a double-blind, randomised, non-inferiority trial. The lancet oncology. 2009 Feb 1; 10(2):135–46.

18. Kubista E, Kenemans P, Foidart JM, Yip CH, Von Schoultz B, Sismondi P, Vassilopoulou-Sellin R, Beckmann MW, Bundred NJ. Safety of tibolone in the treatment of vasomotor symptoms in breast cancer patients—design and baseline data 'LIBERATE' trial. The breast. 2007 Jan 1; 16:182–9.

19. Utian WH, Shoupe D, Bachmann G, Pinkerton JV, Pickar JH. Relief of vasomotor symptoms and vaginal atrophy with lower doses of conjugated equine estrogens and medroxyprogesterone acetate. Fertility and sterility. 2001 Jun 1; 75(6):1065–79.

20. Tan D, Haines CJ, Limpaphayom KK, Holinka CF, Ausmanas MK. Relief of vasomotor symptoms and vaginal atrophy with three doses of conjugated estrogens and medroxyprogesterone acetate in postmenopausal Asian women from 11 countries: The Pan-Asia menopause (PAM) study. Maturitas. 2005 Sep 16; 52(1):35–51.

21. Mosekilde L, Hermann AP, Beck-Nielsen H, Charles P, Nielsen SP, Sørensen OH. The Danish Osteoporosis Prevention Study (DOPS): project design and inclusion of 2000 normal perimenopausal women. Maturitas. 1999 Mar 15; 31(3):207–19.

22. Gierach GL, Johnson BD, Merz CN, Kelsey SF, Bittner V, Olson MB, Shaw LJ, Mankad S, Pepine CJ, Reis SE, Rogers WJ. Hypertension, menopause, and coronary artery disease risk in the Women's Ischemia Syndrome Evaluation (WISE) study. Journal of the American College of Cardiology. 2006 Feb 7; 47(3):S50–8.

23. Sowers MF, Crawford SL, Sternfeld B, Morganstein D, Gold EB, Greendale GA, Evans DA, Neer R, Matthews KA, Sherman S, Lo A. SWAN: a multicenter, multiethnic, community-based cohort study of women and the menopausal transition.

24. Avis NE, Colvin A, Bromberger JT, Hess R, Matthews KA, Ory M, Schocken M. Change in health-related quality of life over the menopausal transition in a multiethnic cohort of middle-aged women: Study of Women's Health Across the Nation (SWAN). Menopause (New York, NY). 2009 Sep; 16(5):860.

25. Matthews KA, Crawford SL, Chae CU, Everson-Rose SA, Sowers MF, Sternfeld B, Sutton-Tyrrell K. Are changes in cardiovascular disease risk factors in midlife women due to chronological aging or to the menopausal transition? Journal of the American College of Cardiology. 2009 Dec 15; 54(25):2366–73.

Self-Assessment

◼ *Punit Bhojani and Deepali Prakash Kale*

1. All of the following are true about estrogen effects except:
   A. Estrogen improves the blood circulation and salt and water content
   B. Estrogen stimulates the cell division of an aging organism
   C. Estrogen stimulates the cell division of mucous membranes
   D. Estrogen inhibits the cell division of supportive and connective tissues

2. According to the 2011 consensus statement what percentage of women contribute to total population of India?
   A. 62%
   B. 70%
   C. 48.46%
   D. None of the above

3. Natural estrogens are:
   A. C 17 compound
   B. C 18 compound
   C. C 19 compound
   D. C 21 compound

4. Premature menopause occurs before the age of:
   A. 40 years
   B. 35 years
   C. 42 years
   D. 45 years

5. 35 years female recently married presented with secondary amenorrhea of 6 months. Pregnancy test is negative. She has irregular periods and only withdrawal bleeding since 1 year. What test confirms premature ovarian insufficiency?
   A. Elevated serum gonadotropins
   B. Elevated serum estradiol
   C. Elevated inhibin B
   D. Atrophic ovaries by transvaginal scan

6. Calcium supplementation is most useful to prevent:
   A. Alzheimer's
   B. Osteoporosis
   C. CVD
   D. Stroke

7. Gynaecological disorder strongly associated with vitamin D deficiency is:
   A. PCOS
   B. Premenstrual syndrome
   C. Uterine fibroids
   D. Endometriosis

8. Analysis of data of women between 50 and 59 years of age in estrogen progesteron therapy arm of WHI trial showed:

A. Increased incidence of venous thromboembolism

B. Increased coronary arterial disease

C. Increased breast cancer incidence

D. None of the above

9. The protein requirements increase in menopause due to which of the following reasons?

A. To help reduce the weight gained

B. To help reduce the effects of muscle loss initiated by the decline in estrogen

C. Both A and B

D. None of the above

10. The hypothesis of 'window of opportunity' developed after:

A. WHI

B. ELITE

C. Nurses health study

D. KEEPS

11. Common side effects of combined MHT all except:

A. Headache

B. Upset stomach, stomach cramps or bloating

C. Diarrhea

D. Appetite and weight changes

E. Changes in sex drive or performance

12. Tibolone has been used for the following indication except:

A. Prevention of postmenopausal osteoporosis

B. Treatment of climacteric symptoms

C. Treatment of postmenopausal osteoporosis

D. Prevention of breast cancer

13. Cystein sulfoxide, (GPCS) that inhibits osteoclast activity is present in:

A. Apple

B. Soya beans

C. Onion

D. Flax seed

14. All of the following are cause of secondary obesity except:

A. Hypothyroidism

B. Insulinoma

C. Diabetes mellitus

D. Cushing's syndrome

15. What are the most commonly followed cut offs for TSH levels internationally?

A. .2–2.5 mIU/L

B. .4–4.5 mIU/L*

C. .1–10 mIU/L

D. None of the above

16. Which is the correct statement about diabetes in menopausal age group:

A. Presence of type 2 diabetes mellitus in women reverses the cardiovascular protective effects of endogenous estrogens before menopause

B. Hyperglycemia and insulin resistance/hyperinsulinemia negate 'estrogen protection' in premenopausal diabetic women

C. None of the above

D. Both A and B are correct

17. Which of the following is true of breast cancer?

A. The lifetime risk for a woman of developing breast cancer is 1/9

B. For most women a specific cause of their breast cancer is known

C. Prognosis is worse for affluent women

D. Incidence of breast cancer is decreasing

18. Fixative for PAP smear is:

A. Normal saline

B. Formaldehyde

C. Alcohol and ether

D. 100% alcohol

19. Simple hyperplasia will progress to Ca endometrium in ____ % of cases

A. 1

B. 5

C. 10

D. 15

20. Which of the following has a normal level of α fetoprotein value in serum?
    A. Ovarian dysgerminoma
    B. Hepatoblastoma
    C. Embryonal carcinoma
    D. Yolk sac tumor

21. European working group on sarcopenia and osteoporosis (EWGSOP) suggests a conceptual staging as:
    A. 'presarcopenia', 'sarcopenia' and 'severe sarcopenia.'
    B. Mild, moderate , severe
    C. Stage I, stage II stage III
    D. Any of the above

22. How much approximately skeletal calcium loss is present when it is picked up by conventional radiography?
    A. 30–40%
    B. 20–30%
    C. 40–50%
    D. 50–60%

23. All of the following are risk factors for osteoporosis except:
    A. Alcohol use
    B. Smoking
    C. Low calcium intake
    D. Obesity
    E. Turner's syndrome

24. All the following are bone resorption markers except:
    A. Hydroxyproline
    B. Pyridinoline and deoxypyridinoline
    C. Bone specific alkaline phosphatase
    D. N telopeptide crosslinks of type I collagen

25. Endometrial hyperplasia associated with granulosa cell tumors is seen in:
    A. 40%
    B. 10%
    C. 20%
    D. 80%

26. 65-year-old female presents with postmenopausal bleeding and the ovarian cystic enlargement on ultra-sonography. Which is the most likely associated ovarian pathology in this condition?
    A. Serous cystadenoma
    B. Mucinous cystadenoma
    C. Granulosa cell tumor
    D. Dermoid cyst

27. Desmopressin is contraindicated in patients with all except:
    A. Renal failure
    B. Hyponatremia
    C. Hypertention
    D. Decreased intracranial pressure

28. Ulipristal is a:
    A. SPRM
    B. SERM
    C. NSAID
    D. Progestin

29. Ulipristol is contraindicated in all except:
    A. Pregnancy
    B. Genital bleeding of undiagnosed etiology
    C. Uterine, cervical, breast cancer
    D. Perimenopausal women

30. A 44-year-old woman presents with menorrhagia but without significant dysmenorrhoea. Given that she wishes to conceive, what would be the best form of treatment?
    A. Tranexamic acid
    B. Etonogestrel implant
    C. Gonadotrophin-releasing hormone agonists
    D. Injected long-acting progestogens
    E. Combined oral contraceptive pill
    F. Levonorgestrel-releasing intra-uterine device
    G. Mefenamic acid
    H. Norethisterone daily from days 5–26 of the cycle

31. Which of the following statements is incorrect regarding levonorgestrel releasing intrauterine system:
    A. There is increased incidence of menorrhagia
    B. This system can be used as hormone replacement therapy
    C. This method is useful for the treatment of endometerial hyperplasia
    D. Irregular uterine bleeding can be problem initially

32. Implanon contains:
    A. Ethinyl estradiol
    B. Etonorgestel
    C. Medroxy progesterone
    D. Gestodene

33. Most common cause of postmenopausal uterine bleeding is:
    A. Endometrial atrophy
    B. Hormone replacement therapy
    C. Endometrial hyperplasia
    D. Endometrial Ca

34. Mrs XY 48-year-old P3L3 is due to undergo a Nova Sure endometrial ablation in theatre for heavy menstrual bleeding, A WHO surgical safety checklist is in progress. Which of the following components of the checklist need to be completed before surgical procedure begins?
    A. Sign in and sign out
    B. Sign in and time in
    C. Sign in and time out
    D. Time in and time out

35. LNG-IUS delivers following amount of levonorgestrel to the endometrium daily:
    A. 20 mcg
    B. 30 mcg
    C. 40 mcg
    D. 50 mcg

36. Which of the following is an indication for endometrial ablation?
    A. Desire for fertility
    B. Young women with a desire to preserve uterus
    C. Endometrial hyperplasia
    D. Postmenopausal women

37. Which surgical procedure has the highest incidence of ureteric injury?
    A. Vaginal hysterectomy
    B. Abdominal hysterectomy
    C. Weitheim's hysterectomy
    D. Anterior colporrhaphy

38. Serum E2 levels after surgical menopause are:
    A. < 10 pg/ml
    B. < 25 pg/ml
    C. ~50 pg/ml
    D. None of the above

39. All of the following are high-risk factors for pelvic organ prolapse except:
    A. Familial and genetic linkage
    B. Smoking
    C. Nulliparity
    D. Menopause

40. The prevalence of pelvic organ prolapse in women over 40 years of age, based solely on patients symptoms ranges from:
    A. 8 to 18%
    B. 0.9 to 3.9%
    C. 2.9 to 8%
    D. 18.3 to 22.3%

41. The term atrophic vaginitis has been replaced by:
    A. Vulvovaginal atrophy
    B. Genitourinary syndrome of menopause
    C. Postmenopausal syndrome
    D. Menopausal atrophy

42. The hypothesis of 'window of opportunity' developed after:
    A. WHI
    B. ELITE
    C. Nurses health study
    D. KEEPS

43. Resistance training has been found associated with all of the following except:
    A. Increased muscle mass
    B. Improved insulin sensitivity
    C. Increased BMI
    D. Increased glucose transport

44. CIN 1 will progress to cancer in __% of cases.
    A. 5
    B. 10

C. < 1
D. 20

45. As per ACOG guidelines, women aged 23 years should have:
    A. PAP test every 5 years
    B. PAP test every 3 years
    C. No need for PAP test
    D. PAP test and HPV testing every 2 years

Answer Key

1. D	10. D	19. A	28. A	37. C
2. C	11. E	20. A	29. D	38. A
3. A	12. D	21. A	30. A	39. C
4. A	13. C	22. A	31. A	40. C
5. A	14. C	23. D	32. B	41. B
6. B	15. B	24. C	33. A	42. A
7. A	16. D	25. A	34. C	43. C
8. A	17. A	26. C	35. A	44. C
9. C	18. C	27. D	36. B	45. D